CURRENT PERSPECTIVES ON LESS-KNOWN ASPECTS OF HEADACHE

Edited by **Hande Turker**

Current Perspectives on Less-known Aspects of Headache
http://dx.doi.org/10.5772/62616
Edited by Hande Turker

Contributors
Edoardo Raposio, Francesco Simonacci, Nicolò Bertozzi, Chiara Bordin, Tuba Edgünlü, Sevim Karakaş Çelik, Birte Tornøe, Yasushi Shibata, Sumire Chiku, Sertaç Argun Kıvanç, Berna Akova-Budak, Mahmut Oğuz Ulusoy, Osman Okan Olcaysü, Nilüfer Yeşilırmak, Bardia Amirlak, Xingchen Li, Kyle Sanniec, Michael Chung, Daniela Matei, Dan Cuciureanu, Irina Constantinescu, Victor Constantinescu, Müge Güler Özden

Published by InTech
Janeza Trdine 9, 51000 Rijeka, Croatia

Publishing Process Manager Martina Usljebrka
Technical Editor SPi Global
Cover InTech Design team

First published April, 2017
Printed in Croatia
Legal deposit, Croatia: National and University Library in Zagreb

Additional hard copies can be obtained from orders@intechopen.com

Current Perspectives on Less-known Aspects of Headache, Edited by Hande Turker
p. cm.
Print ISBN 978-953-51-3075-8
Online ISBN 978-953-51-3076-5

For EU product safety concerns:
IN TECH d.o.o., Prolaz Marije Krucifikse Kozulić 3, 51000 Rijeka, Croatia,
info@intechopen.com or visit our website at intechopen.com.

Meet the editor

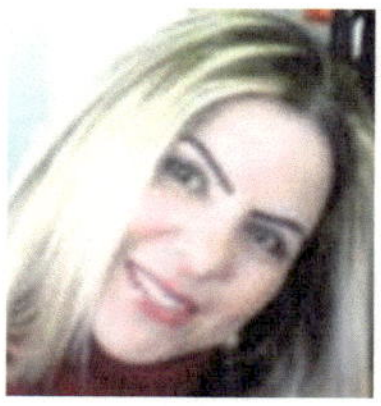

Hande Turker is a neurologist and a clinical neurophysiologist. She has been dealing with headache, neuropathic pain, neuromuscular diseases, dystonia, and electromyography and evoked potentials for nearly 25 years. She is the author of many publications including several book chapters on evoked potentials and electromyography. Her main interests other than clinical neurophysiology are neuropathic pain, headache, and botulinum toxin injections in movement disorders. She has been working at Ondokuz Mayıs University, Samsun, Turkey, since 2003. She is an associate professor and lecturer and teaches headache, neuropathic pain, neuromuscular diseases, and electromyography and evoked potentials at the university where she founded the "Evoked Potential Lab" and directed the EMG and EP Unit between 2003 and 2010.
She is also the author of InTech book chapters "*Middle and Long Latency Auditory Evoked Potentials and Their Usage in Fibromyalgia and Schizophrenia*," "**N***eurological Complications of Hypothyroidism*," and "*Surface Electromyography in Sports and Exercise*." She is the editor of the InTech book *Electrodiagnosis in New Frontiers of Clinical Research*.

Contents

Preface IX

Section 1 Pathophysiology, Diagnosis and Differential Diagnosis of Headache 1

Chapter 1 **Genetic Aspect of Headache 3**
Tuba Gökdoğan Edgünlü and Sevim Karakas Çelik

Chapter 2 **Children and Adolescents with Primary Tension-Type Headaches: Research and Practice Perspectives for Non-Pharmacological Interdisciplinary Headache Service 25**
Birte Tornøe

Chapter 3 **Primary Headaches and their Relationship with the Autonomic Nervous System 45**
Cuciureanu Dan Iulian, Constantinescu Irina, Constantinescu Victor, Corciova Calin and Matei Daniela

Chapter 4 **Relation between Smartphone Use and Unilateral Ocular Pain and Headache 77**
Sertaç Argun Kıvanç, Berna Akova Budak, Mahmut Oğuz Ulusoy, Osman Okan Olcaysü and Nilüfer Yeşilırmak

Chapter 5 **Trichodynia (Scalp Dysesthesia) 85**
Müge Güler Özden

Section 2 Therapeutical Aspects in Headache 91

Chapter 6 **Surgical Therapy of Migraine and Tension-Type Headache 93**
Edoardo Raposio, Nicolò Bertozzi, Chiara Bordin and Francesco Simonacci

Chapter 7 **Surgical Management of Migraine Headaches 115**
Michael Chung, Kyle Sanniec, Xingchen Li and Bardia Amirlak

Chapter 8 **Management of Migraine Headaches: OnabotulinumtoxinA Injection 129**
Michael Chung, Xingchen Li, Kyle Sanniec and Bardia Amirlak

Chapter 9 **Acupuncture as a Therapy for Headache 145**
Sumire Chiku and Yasushi Shibata

Preface

When I first accepted to edit this book you will read, I did not quite imagine that the content would be about so many less-known and "still containing question marks" subjects about headache. As time passed and more submitted chapters came along, I realized that most of the chapters composing this book contained many answers to many unanswered questions about headache in general.

Headache, as a main neurological problem in everyday life, still takes place as a contributor on top of the list of many partially solved neurological conditions. Not only primary headaches but secondary headaches are still clinical concerns of diagnosis, differential diagnosis, and therapy.

As a neurologist who has been seeing headache patients for 25 years, I made a simple list of questions about headache that are often asked by my students, residents, patients, and colleagues so far and tried to find some interesting ones among them. The objective results about my "self-questionnaire" did indeed surprise me! The content in the book did not answer all but answered most of them, for example, "Is headache a genetic condition?", "What do smartphones do to our brains? Do they cause headaches?", and "Does botulinum toxin really improve chronic migraine?". The examples may be increased of course.

This book is quite different from classical headache books. First of all, it does not contain the classical schema of a classical headache textbook. The most important answer for the reason is that the need for non–textbook-type medical books is increasing as the needs of medical doctors in the field are changing from day to day.

In the first section of this book, you will recognize interesting chapters about pathophysiology, diagnosis, and differential diagnosis about some headache types. In the second section, mostly nonpharmacological therapeutic aspects of headache are discussed in the chapters, and some chapters are written by nonneurologist specialists. This should not, however, raise frowns among neurologists. We neurologists believe that headache patients should be seen by neurologists first, especially for the first diagnosis, but other specialists may contribute when necessary. General practitioners and family doctors see headache patients, and the number of patients they see may surprise so many people.

I hope and believe this book will be an interesting read and perhaps a guide in some new aspects of headache and help understand "some interesting headache issues" while stressing the less known mentioned above.

I thank all the authors of the book without whom this book would not be published. I will also thank my colleague and mentor who inspired me, Prof. Dr. Taner Özbenli, an important name in headache.

Finally, I dedicate this book to my headache patients, my students, residents, and all my mentors from whom I have learned so much.

Assoc. Prof. Dr. Hande Turker, MD, MS
Neurologist and Clinical Neurophysiologist
Ondokuz Mayıs University, Department of Neurology, School of Medicine
Samsun, Turkey

Section 1

Pathophysiology, Diagnosis and Differential Diagnosis of Headache

Chapter 1

Genetic Aspect of Headache

Tuba Gökdoğan Edgünlü and Sevim Karakas Çelik

Additional information is available at the end of the chapter

http://dx.doi.org/10.5772/66852

Abstract

Headache is a multifactorial disease and the genetic basis is not clear yet. We review recent findings about molecular basis of subtypes of headache. The fundamentals of molecular genetics and the recent advances in this area are important for clinicians to understand the pathogenesis of the disorder. Recent studies provide a foundation for critical appraisal of the literature, unprecedented insights and reveal promising treatment targets for future drug development. This chapter provides an overview of molecular genetics, epigenetic and genome-wide association studies on headache. In summary, we try to explain the state-of-the-art molecular basis of headache and the possible future direction in this field of research studies. According to recent studies the main types of are evaluative, exploratory about molecular basis of headache. In recent years, new studies have been designed to provide an update and understanding of the modern day genetics, the advances in genetic research and methods and a basis for understanding the strategy by which advances in molecular genetics can be applied for understanding complex polygenetic diseases such as migraine.

Keywords: headache, genetic, epigenetic, cluster type headache, tension type headache, migraine

1. Molecular basis of headache subtypes

Recently, researchers have identified the gene variations that increase the susceptibility to develop headaches. To analyze the cause, clinical history of headaches is very important. While headaches can be caused by medical conditions, injuries, or infections, sometimes they are not due to any specific disease or other identified medical conditions. The three most common of those types of primary headaches are tension, cluster and migraine headaches (**Figure 1**). Tension-type headache (TTH) brought on by stress or depression, so everyone has

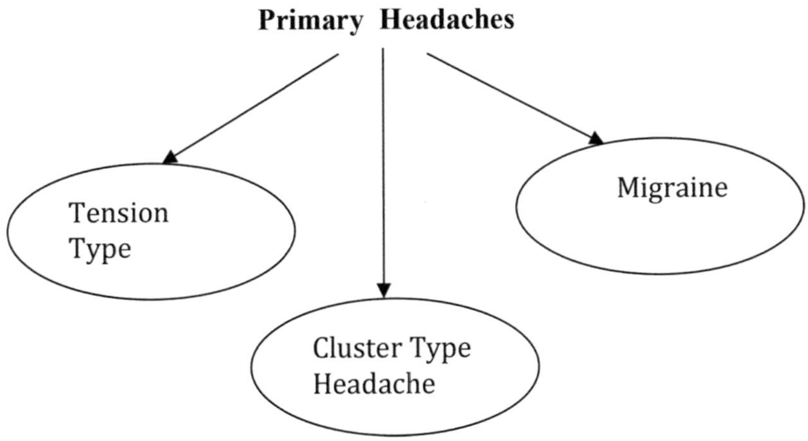

Figure 1. Diagram of primary headaches subtypes.

experienced TTH. TTH can be brief, episodic or continuous. According to some researchers, TTH could be secondary to the vasoconstriction, rather than dilatation [1–3].

The neurobiological mechanisms of tension-type headache are concerning. Central sensitization plays a major role in chronic TTH. Whether peripheral mechanisms or central mechanisms are primarily responsible for TTH is an important issue to differentiate it pathophysiologically from migraine. The literature suggests that migraine and tension-type headache may have the similar pathophysiology. Moreover, exact mechanism for both the disorders is still to be elucidated [4–6].

The prevalence of migraine has been shown to be increasing. The researchers have suggested that the central nervous system (CNS) susceptible to headache has been linked to an important survival or reproductive advantage. Some possible reasons are determined; one of these says that migraine is a defense mechanism; the other one consider it as a result of novel environmental factors; the next one regards migraine as a compromise between genetic harms and benefits. Genetic epidemiological studies are necessary to prove the involvement of genetic factors. Twin studies have been used to assess the respective roles of genetic and environmental factors in migraine [7, 8].

We briefly mention here the headache types and characteristics. The first title is TTH. Biological mechanisms of TTH are yet to be explained. This disease usually is associated with depression and anxiety. In addition, the genetic factors are most important for TTH pathogenesis. The neurological mechanisms of TTH are not known clearly. Genetic and neurobiological research studies have increased our understanding of the complex mechanisms that may lead to TTH. There is strong evidence for a genetic predisposition for TTH. Moreover pain pathways in the central nervous system are positively associated with TTH. Research has enhanced our current understanding regarding the means through which psychological factors lead to TTH, suggesting sympathetic hyperactivity as a possible mechanism [9, 10].

The etiology of cluster-type headache (CH) is still unknown. Until recently, researchers thought that CH was not an inherited disorder; however, several new studies have suggested that genetic factors play an important role in the CH. Some studies show that CH phenotype is inherited such as in autosomal dominant disease [11, 12]

To identify genetic factors that confer susceptibility to migraine, many studies have been conducted on the genetic basis of migraine types. First approach on this is classical linkage analysis. This approach aims to identify affected segments of chromosomes in individuals using a family-based approach. For monogenic migraine types, this approach has been particularly successful. A second commonly used strategy to identify gene variants involves candidate-gene association studies. These studies are determinate with alleles and genotype frequencies in control and case groups. Recently, DNA variants have advanced spectacularly, allowing the cost-effective analysis of DNA variants in patients in so-called genome-wide association studies (GWAS). Also, GWAS included hundreds of genes for many complex diseases. To determine the size of rarer gene variants is too expensive and takes more time. Instead, methods such as next-generation sequencing of exons (exome sequencing) and whole-genome sequencing can be used [13].

2. Genetic aspects of tension-type headache

While tension-type headaches (TTH) are the most common primary headache disorder it has not been as thoroughly investigated as migraine headaches. A lifetime prevalence of TTH has been seen in the general population ranging between 30 and 78% in different studies [13]. Nevertheless, 24–37% had TTH several times a month, 10% had it weekly and 2–3% of the population had chronic TTH, usually lasting for the greater part of their lifetime [14] According to the second edition of the International Classification of Headache Disorders, TTH is classified into three subtypes according to headache frequency: infrequent episodic TTH, frequent episodic TTH and chronic TTH [13]. The female-to-male ratio of TTH is 5:4 indicating that, unlike migraine, women are affected only slightly more than men [15]. The average age of onset of TTH is higher than in migraine, namely 25 to 30 years in cross-sectional epidemiologic studies [16].

Many studies probably provide a valid measure of the major etiologic role that genetic or environmental factors play in TTH. **Table 1** shows the genetic association studies in TTH. In a study of twins from the New Danish Twin Registry, it was found that the concordance rates were significantly higher in MZ than same-gender DZ twin pairs with no or frequent episodic TTH, while the difference was not significant in chronic TTH due to small number of twin pairs. In monozygotic (MZ) and same-gender DZ twin pairs, the concordance rates of infrequent episodic tension-type headache was significantly different in women but not in men, although the difference was small in both genders. It was suggested that genetic factors play a role in no and frequent episodic tension-type headache, while infrequent episodic TTH is caused primarily by environmental factors [17]. However, differently Ulrich et al. suggested that an environmental influence was of major importance for episodic TTH and a genetic factor had minor contribution [18] but in chronic tension-type headache, the genetic factor may be more important.

When the population-relative risk in first- degree relatives compared with normal controls has been calculated in a Danish study, it was shown that first-degree relatives of 122 probands with chronic tension headache had more than three times the risk of chronic tension

Gene	Genetic variants	Results	Reference
Monoamine oxidase (MAO)	rs1799836 G/A promoter polymorphism of a variable number of tandem repeats (VNTR)	No association	[21]
Catechol-O-methyltransferase (COMT)	Val158Met	may be involved in the phenotypic expression	[25]
Tumor necrosis factor (TNF)	TNFA 308G > A and TNFB 252G > A	No association	[40]
Estrogen receptor (ESR1) progesterone receptor (PROGINS)	ESR1 PvuII (rs2234693), ESR1 325 C→G (rs1801132)] and [(rs1042838)	No association	[119]
Apolipoprotein E (APOE)		Association	[28]
Serotonin (5-hydroxytryptamine, 5HT) transporter gene	the variable number of tandem repeats (VNTR) and 5'-flanking promoter region (5-HTTLPR)	Association	[33]
Serotonin transporter gene	5-HTTLPR)	Association	[34]
Serotonin transporter gene	5-HTTLPR	Association	[35]
Serotonin transporter gene	5HTR2c-Cys23Ser	No association	[36]
Glutathione S-transferase (GST) M1, T1, P1	GST M1 and T1 null polymorphism GSTP1 $Ile^{105}Val$	No Association	[42]
Methylenetetrahydrofolate reductase gene (MTHFR)	C677T and A1298C	Association	[38]
Methylenetetrahydrofolate reductase gene (MTHFR)	C677T	No association	[39]

Table 1. The genetic association studies in TTH.

headache than the general population. An increased family risk can be caused by genetic or environmental factors because probands and spouses share their environment, the risk of chronic tension headache in spouses is used to elucidate the relative role of genetic and environmental factors. As first-degree relatives had a significantly increased risk of chronic tension headache and spouses had no increased risk, this result supports the importance of genetic factors in chronic tension headache. [19]. For investigation of the mode of inheritance of chronic tension-type headache complex segregation analysis was performed in 122 Danish families. The complex segregation analysis indicates that chronic tension-type headache has multifactorial inheritance [20].

Because TTH treatment features medication with inhibitors for selective reuptake of serotonin and monoamine oxidase inhibitors, The polymorphic patterns of MAOA and MAOB, both in TTH patients and the healthy population were addressed in our previous study. MAO gene polymorphisms were examined in a group of 120 TTH patients and in another 168 unrelated healthy volunteers (control group). MAOA promoter and MAOB intron 13 polymorphisms were genotyped using PCR-based methods. But an overall comparison between genotype and allele frequencies of the patients and the control group did not reveal any statistically significant difference between the patients and the control group [21].

The catechol-O-methyltransferase (COMT) is an enzyme involved in the metabolic degradation of dopamine, norepinephrin and epinephrine [22]. It is accepted that COMT gene is one of the several potential headache genetic determinants. Several studies indicate that the genetic polymorphism due to a G→A substitution at codon 158 of the COMT gene, which leads to the formation of a heat-stable, high-activity COMT variant (Val/Val) and heat-labile, low-activity variants (Val/Met or Met/Met) [23]. Zubieta et al. demonstrated that a measure of pain sensitivity paralleled the COMT activity of the genotypes and individuals with Val/Val genotype have reduced pain sensitivity compared with those with the Met/Met genotype [24]. And also, Fernández-de-las-Peñas C et al. investigate the relationship between Val158Met polymorphisms, headache and pressure hypersensitivity in children with chronic tension-type headache (CTTH). But it was reported that the Val158Met COMT polymorphism does not appear to be involved in predisposition to suffer from CTTH in children; nevertheless, this genetic factor may be involved in the phenotypic expression, as pressure hypersensitivity was greater in those CTTH children with the Met/Met genotype [25]. Nitric oxide has an important role in the pathophysiology of tension-type headache. It is suggested nitric oxide synthetase inhibitors are helpful in the management of chronic tension-type headache by reducing the central sensitization [26]. Besides nitric oxide synthetase, nitric oxide production is also dependent on apolipoprotein E (APOE) polymorphism and this production is gene specific [27]. And it was investigated that APOE polymorphism may be associated with migraine as well as tension-type headache. And the results of the study showed that APOE epsilon2 gene increases the risk of migraine, while APOE epsilon4 gene is protective against migraine and tension-type headache [28].

As other neurotransmitters, serotonin have a role in pain mechanisms, selective serotonin re-uptake inhibitors (SSRIs) reduce the symptomatic/analgesic medication use for acute headache attacks of tension-type headache [29]. Serotonin is taken up from the synaptic space regularly with a 5-hydroxytryptamine transporter (5-HTT) [30, 31]. Two polymorphic sites in 5-HTT gene was studied in various studies: different numbers of variable-number-tandem-repeat (VNTR) region of 16-17 base-pair (bp) in the second intron of 5-HTT gene leads several alleles such as STin 2.7, STin 2.9, STin 2.10, STin 2.11, STin 2.12 and a 44-base pair insertion/deletion in the 5'--flanking promoter region (5-HTT gene-linked polymorphic region-5-HTTLPR) creating a short (S) and a long (L) allele [32]. The possible role of 5-HTTLPR and VNTR polymorphisms was evaluated individually and in combination in risk of CTTH. Moreover, the relationship between the clinical response of the drugs or analgesic overuse and the serotonin transporter (5-HTT) gene polymorphisms was investigated [33, 34]. Park et al. reported that S/S genotype frequency was significantly higher in patients with CTH (76%) than in those with controls (59%; P =.02). The authors suggested that 5-HTTLPR might be one of the genetically contributing factors [35].

But differently in another study any statistically significant results based on the 5-HTTLPR gene alleles and CTTH risk were not found. Only, when it was investigated the combined effect of the two polymorphic loci of the 5-HTT gene, genotypes S/S-12/10 and L/S-12/10 displayed statistically significant frequency in the CTTH group than in the control group. Aylin et al. reported that the presence of homozygous L and STin12 alleles may play a protective role against CTTH [33]. Also in a different study showed that the S/S genotype frequency was significantly higher in CTTH patients with analgesic overuse. And it was suggested that serotonergic activity may be involved in the development of analgesic overuse in CTTH and that 5-HTTLPR might be one of the genetically contributing factors [34]. But no significant differences were noticed between the 5-HTTLPR and VNTR haplotype groups and success in treatment. 5HT2c-receptor (5HTR2c) is another subtypes of 5HT2 families. The relationship between 5HTR2c Cys23Ser polymorphism and TTH was also investigated. However, there were no differences found among TTH and control groups [36].

Increased homocysteine levels are associated with various pathological conditions in humans, including stroke and cardiovascular disorders. So vasodilation of cerebral blood vessels may result in headache, or high levels of homocysteine may cause temporary thrombosis of cerebral blood vessels, allowing less oxygen into the brain thus possibly causing headache. Frosst et al. reported an association between the homozygous C677T mutation in the 5,10-methylenetetrahydrofolate reductase (MTHFR) gene and serum homocysteine levels [37]. In a case-control study, the prevalence of two common MTHFR polymorphisms, C677T and A1298C, in tension-type headache patients and healthy controls was compared. And it was suggested that patients with C1298C and C677C/C1298C genotypes may predispose to tension-type headache [38]. On the contrary, the study of Kowa et al. could not reach the same results. It was reported that MTHFR gene polymorphisms was not a genetic risk factor for TTH in their study [39].

Also it was investigated the relationship between TTH and tumor necrosis factor (TNF) gene polymorphisms (TNFA 308G > A and TNFB 252G > A) [40] and also estrogen receptor [ESR1 PvuII (rs2234693), ESR1 325 C→G (rs1801132)] and progesterone receptor [PROGINS (rs1042838)] polymorphisms [41]. But no risk was observed when TTH patients were compared with HC. Similarly, in a study that evaluates the relationship between GSTM1, T1 and P1 gene polymorphism and TTH, no difference was found between two groups in the genotype and allele distribution [42].

3. Genetic aspects of cluster-type headache

Cluster headache (CH), the most severe primary headache, is characterized by recurrent, unilateral attacks of headache of great intensity and brief duration, accompanied by local signs and symptoms of autonomic dysfunction. In about 80% of the patients, the attacks occur in series lasting weeks or months, so-called cluster periods [3]. The disease has an estimated prevalence of 1/500 and displays marked sex bias (female:male ratio 1:2.5 to 1:3.5) [43, 44].

Twin studies represent one of the simplest ways to unravel the relative importance of genetic and environmental effects. Much of the available literature on CH is reported in numerous concordant monozygotic twin pairs [45–48]. However, other studies demonstrated discordant twin pairs showed the importance of both genetic and individual specific factors and environmental factors in CH [49]. Beside this, epidemiological surveys indicate that compared with the general population, the first-degree relatives of CH patients had a 14 fold increase in the disease risk in affected Danish probands and 39 fold increase in affected Italian probands.

Also second-degree relatives have two times higher risk in Danish probands and eight times higher risk in Italian probands [50–52]. The different results can be partly explained by methodological differences or selection bias. The increased familial risk of CH strongly suggests a genetic cause for the disease. However, the pattern of inheritance does not appear to be uniform. The familial clustering supports a model of autosomal dominant inheritance with reduced penetrance in some families but autosomal recessive model in others [53, 54] Also a study by Sjöstrand demonstrated a significantly lower mean age of onset in the second/third generation of families with CH than in the first generation. This can be explained by anticipation or selection bias, since individuals with late age at onset from the second/third generation may not yet have symptoms [55, 56].

To date, no clear molecular genetic evidence has been shown for CH. A point mutation was reported in mitochondrial transfer RNAleu(UUR) gene at nucleotide pair 3243 in a Japanese man with sporadic CH [56]. However, this mutation was not detected in Italian and German patients with CH [57, 58] and the involvement of mitochondrial genes in CH remains unproven.

Neuroimaging studies have identified the posterolateral hypothalamic grey matter as the key area for the basic defect in CH [59]. Hypocretin-1 and -2 (also called orexin-A and -B) are newly discovered neuropeptides [60, 61]. Hypocretin-containing cells are located exclusively in the posterolateral hypothalamus, with widespread projections to the entire neuroaxis. Hypocretin-1 and -2 bind to 2 G protein-coupled receptors, termed HCRTR1 and HCRTR2. The peptides of the hypocretin/orexin system influence a wide range of physiologic and behavioral processes in mammals [62, 63]. Some of these, such as sleep, neuroendocrine, locomotor, autonomic regulation, feeding behavior and energy homeostasis, may be of relevance for the pathogenesis of CH. Also a striking feature of CH is its diurnal and seasonal periodicity, suggesting that circadian and infradian rhythms regulate CH attacks. The hypocretin system plays a pivotal role in generating such rhythms and hypocretin-containing neurons originate almost exclusively from the posterolateral hypothalamus [60, 61, 64]. Recent studies suggest a contribution of hypocretin to the pathogenesis of CH. A study among 109 Italian CH patients showed a strong association between the hypocretin type 2 receptor (HCRTR2) G1246A polymorphism and CH [65]. This association was confirmed in a major study from Germany, showing that homozygous carriers of the G-allele had a twofold increase in disease risk [66]. Also in another study among Italian patients five additional intronic polymorphisms was genotyped, covering more than 75% of the entire 108.35 kb sequence of the HCRTR2 gene. And the carriage of the GTAAGG haplotype was shown to be associated with the disease and resulted in a 3.7-fold increased risk for CH [67]. On the contrary, the association was not replicated in a dataset of CH patients of Danish, Swedish and British origin [68]. In addition there are two published meta-analysis studies investigating the association between polymorphisms of the HCRTR2 gene and CH. However, there are conflicting results between two studies, Rainero et al. suggested that the G1246A polymorphism of the HCRTR2 gene may modulate the genetic risk for CH [69] but Weller et al. did not find evidence for association of G1246A polymorphism (rs2653349) [70].

Besides this, the association between CH and a variable number tandem repeat (VNTR) polymorphism of the PER3 clock gene that has been associated to preferred daily rhythm (chronotype) in several studies was investigated. The hypothalamic biological clock may thus be involved in the pathophysiology and 149 patients were genotyped, but no difference in PER3 VNTR polymorphisms between patients and controls was found. And no association between CH, PER3 VNTR polymorphism and chronotype was found in the study [71].

Also some researchers performed a genetic association study to evaluate the relationship between CH and polymorphisms in the Clock gene, another highly conserved circadian gene, that influence the circadian phase in humans [72]. But they found that phenotype and allele frequencies were similarly distributed in CH patients and controls. Also it was determined that the clinical features of the disease were not significantly influenced by different genotypes. In conclusion, studies reported that the 3092 T-->C polymorphism of the Clock gene is unlikely to play an important role in CH [73, 74].

Recent studies suggested that iron metabolism may be involved in the pathophysiology of primary headaches. The genetic association studies are shown in **Table 2**. In patients with migraine and chronic daily headache, Welch and colleagues [75] reported elevated iron concentrations in the periaqueductal gray matter, one of the pain-modulating centers of the brainstem. To evaluate whether mutations of the HFE gene would modify the occurrence and the clinical features of CH, an association study was performed in a cohort of Italian CH patients and healthy controls. They did not find C282Y mutation in both controls and cases. The prevalence of the H63D mutation was nearly similar in controls and cases so it was suggested that genetic variations within the HFE gene are associated with CH. But the HFE D63D genotype determined showed the onset of the disease at a significantly later age in comparison with both H63H and H63D patients. So they recommended the HFE gene may influence the disease phenotype and may be regarded as a disease modifier gene [76].

Nitric oxide (NO) plays a critical role in the regulation of vasodilation, neurotransmission, inflammation and many other events throughout the body. NO also appears to be an important mediator of vascular headache pathophysiology [77, 78]. And an association analysis of five polymorphic microsatellite markers in the three different NO synthase (NOS) genes; nNOS (NOS1), iNOS (NOS2A) and eNOS (NOS3) was performed. However, it is unlikely that genetic variations within the NOS genes contribute greatly to CH susceptibility [79].

Methylenetetrahydrofolate reductase (MTHFR) is a key enzyme in the remethylation pathway converting homocysteine to methionine. The TT genotype of the common MTHFR 677C>T polymorphism (rs1801133) has been shown to impair enzyme activity and increase homocysteine levels [37]. It was shown that this variant has been linked to migraine in recent meta-analyses [80, 81] Homocysteine and oxidized metabolites like homocysteic acid exert excitatory effects on neurons and homocysteic acid has been shown to increase cell firing of trigeminal neurons [82]. Hence, a link between the MTHFR 677C>T polymorphism and CH is plausible. But in an investigation on the association between the MTHFR 677C>T polymorphism and CH among German patients and controls do not indicate an association between genotypes of the MTHFR 677C>T polymorphism and CH overall [83].

Alcohol is a well-known trigger factor for CH attacks during the active phases of the disease. The alcohol dehydrogenase (ADH) pathway, which converts alcohol to the toxic substance

Gene	Genetic variants	Results	Reference
Alcohol dehydrogenase 4 (ADH4)	rs1800759 (-136AC) rs1126671 (Ile328Val)	No association	[85]
Period (PER3)	VNTR polymorphism	No association	[71]
Hypocretin receptor 2 (HCRTR2)	G1246A (rs2653349)	No association	[70]
5-HTTLPR	rs4795541 (3-bp insdel) rs25531 (A > G)	No association	
Alcohol dehydrogenase (ADH4)	rs1800759 (-136AC) rs1126671 (Ile328Val)	Association	[84]
Methylenetetrahydrofolate reductase gene (MTHFR)	rs1801133 (677C>T)	No association	[83]
Hypocretin Receptor-2 (HCRTR2)	Haplotype of rs10498801, rs3122156, rs9357855, rs2653342, rs3800539, rs2653349	Association	[67]
CLOCK Gene	rs1801260 (T3092C)	No association	[73]
HCRTR2	G1246A (rs2653349)	Association	[69]
HCRTR2	G1246A (rs2653349)	No association with drug responses in CH	
G protein beta3 subunit	rs5443 (C825T)	Association with triptan response	[87]
Hypocretin receptor 2 (HCRTR2)	G1246A (rs2653349)	Association	
Clock gene	rs1801260 (T3092C)	No association	[76]
Calcium channel gene (CACNA1A)	SSCP analysis of all 47 exons	No association	[89]
Calcium channel gene (CACNA1A)		No association	[88]
HFE (hemochromatosis)	C282Y and H63D	No association	[76]
Hypocretin (HCRT) Hypocretin receptor (HCRTR1) Hypocretin receptor 2 (HCRTR2)	-3250CT rs8072081 (-1717CT) rs1056526 (T264C) rs2271933 (C1375T) rs2653349 (G1246A) rs1027650 (IVS4 12.564AC)	Not polymorphic Not polymorphic No association No association Association No association	[65]

Table 2. The genetic association studies in CH.

acetaldehyde, is responsible for most of the alcohol breakdown in the liver. And Rainero and colleagues investigated the association of genetic variants within the ADH4 gene with CH susceptibility and phenotype. They suggested that CH was associated with the ADH4 gene or a linked locus. For rs1126671 polymorphism, the carriage of the AA genotype, in comparison with remaining genotypes, was associated with a significantly increased disease risk of 2.33 times. [84] But the results were not confirmed in Swedish population. The data from this study did not support an association of the ADH4 SNPs rs1126671 and rs1800759 with CH [85].

Only about 70% of migraine and CH patients report significant treatment responses to triptans, which are agonists at 5-HT1B/D receptors belonging to the family of G protein-coupled receptors. A C825T polymorphism identified in the gene for the G protein β3 (Gβ3) subunit (GNB3) has been associated with an enhanced signal transduction via GPCR [86]. It was investigated whether a common polymorphism in the gene for the G protein β3 subunit (GNB3 C825T) modulates responder rates to triptans among a large cohort of Caucasian CH patients. It was suggested that pain relief by triptans is significantly modulated by a common genetic GNB3 variant [88].

Also mutations of the P/Q type calcium channel alpha 1 subunit (CACNA1A) gene on chromosome 19p13 have been shown to cause several neurological disorders with a wide clinical spectrum, mainly episodic diseases. Missense mutations of the gene cause familial hemiplegic migraine (FHM) and it is also likely to be involved in the more common forms of migraine. It was investigated whether the CACNA1A gene is also a candidate gene for CH. In this study an association analysis of an intragenic polymorphic (CA)n-repeat with marker D19S1150 and a (CAG)n-repeat in the 3'UTR region was performed, in 75 patients with CH in Swedish population. But it was found that genotypes and allele frequencies were similarly distributed in patients and controls. Also linkage disequilibrium between the two markers was similar in patients and controls. And it was suggested that any significance of the CACNA1A gene in CH is unlikely [88]. Similarly Haan J et al. suggested that there is no involvement of the calcium channel gene (CACNA1A) mutations in a Dutch family with CH [89].

4. Genetic aspect of migraine

Migraine is an episodic and disabling neurological disorder affecting roughly 14% of the population. The two most prevalent forms are migraine without aura (MO) and migraine with aura (MA). Migraine tends to run in families and has a strong genetic basis, with heritability estimates of 40–57%. In the rare monogenic subtype of migraine, familial hemiplegic migraine (FHM), three causative genes have been identified. There is, however, no significant association between these genes and MO and/or MA. Many linkage studies and candidate gene studies have suggested causative genes in MO and MA, but few have been replicated. Recent attempts using genome-wide association studies (GWAS) have yielded four single nucleotide polymorphisms (SNPs) that are significantly associated with migraine and recently, three additional SNPs have shown convincing association as well [90–93].

Recently, several studies have been used to identify genetic variants either causing migraine or conferring vulnerability to the disease. The array-based technologies and second-generation DNA sequencing has provided novel analysis to genetic database. In general, rare variants are sought by DNA sequencing in multigenerational families with many affected individuals. These studies were previously performed using a linkage approach, followed by refinement of the linkage region and targeted Sanger sequencing of candidate genes. On the other hand, genome-wide association studies (GWAS) allowed the determination of the case-control or family-based association studies in large samples [93].

Many studies are conducted for understanding of molecular genetic basis of MA, MO and FHM well. Especially GWAS has given very important results for these diseases. The present work does not represent a systematic review but rather aims to provide thorough coverage of this area of investigation. Migraine can be part of known genetic disorders, displaying multiple manifestations and often involving various organs.

Migraine is associated with some of genetic syndromes. These diseases are CADASIL cerebral autosomal dominant arteriopathy with subcortical infarcts and leukoencephalopathy, COL4A1 retinal arteriolar tortuosity and leukoencephalopathy, CRV cerebroretinal vasculopathy, CSD cortical spreading depression, FASPS familial anticipated sleep phase syndrome, HERNS hereditary endotheliopathy with retinopathy, nephropathy, stroke, HVR hereditary vascular retinopathy, MELAS mitochondrial encephalomyopathy, lactic acidosis, stroke-like episodes, RVCL retinal vasculopathy and cerebral leukodystrophy These disorders, though rare, may lead to a better comprehension of the mechanisms underlying more common forms of idiopathic migraine. Other forms of typical FHM due to mutations in novel FHM candidate genes have been recently described. Mutations resulting in an FHM phenotype have been identified in the PRRT2 (proline-rich transmembrane protein 2) gene, located on human chromosome 16p11 and encoding for an axonal protein associated with the exocytosis protein complex [94–99].

Studies shown that FHM is related to CACNA1A gene which encoded by 19p13, which produces voltage-dependent (P/Q) Cav 2.1 channel, α1A subunit Over 70 missense mutations with "gain of function" effect. ATP1A2 encoded by 1q21-23 that produce to Na^+-K^+ ATPase α2 subunit responsible for FHM 2 disease. FHM3 is related to SCN1A gene. In conclusion, familial forms of MA and in particular FHM, are due to rare inherited or sporadic genetic variants endowed with high penetrance. These mutations are affecting the transmembrane electrochemical gradient by enhancing extracellular glutamate concentrations which are related with neuronal excitability [100, 101]. We can explain migraine-associated genes in four groups and other effective mechanisms (**Figure 2**).

4.1. Candidate genes

(1) Neurological genes: This group candidate genes encode (a)ion channels (calcium channel, voltage-dependent, P/Q type, alpha 1A subunit [CACNA1A], voltage-potassium intermediate/small conductance calcium-activated channel and subfamily N, member 3 [KCCN3]) (b) Na+/K+-ATPase subunits, (c) molecules involved in the synthesis, release and binding of neuropeptides (calcitonin gene-related peptide) or neurotransmitters (glutamate, GABA, dopamine, serotonin) relevant to neuronal excitation and/or to nociception. Some case-control association studies have yielded positive results, as known 5-HT-related genes, MAOA, dopamine-related genes, although most studies have been negative especially for the former two

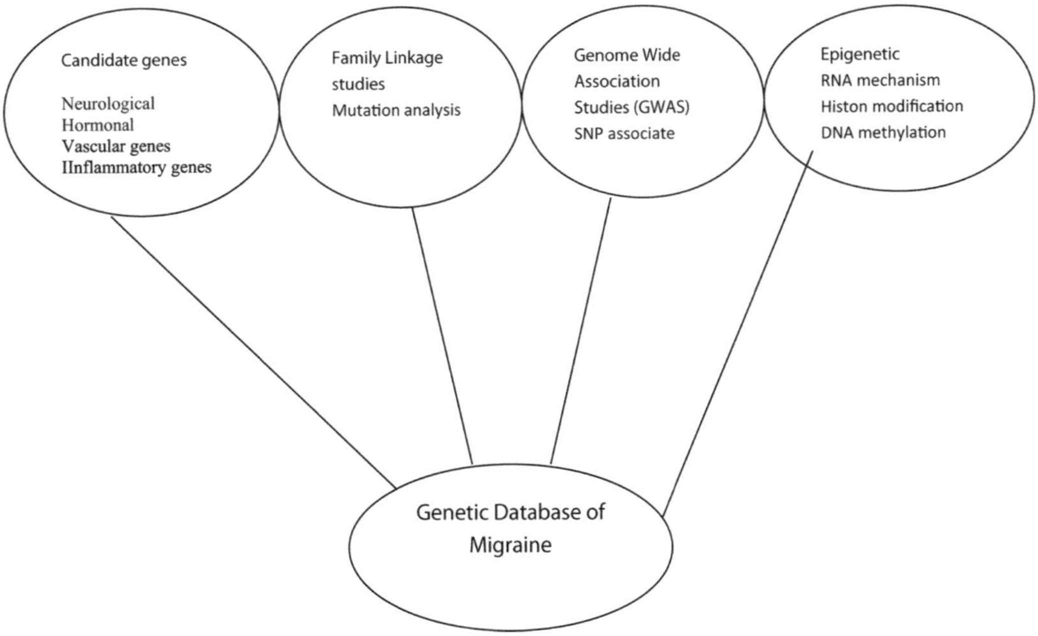

Figure 2. Genetic database of migraine disease.

gene families. Nonetheless, a thorough screening of 150 brain-expressed genes involved in ion homeostasis (channels, transporters, exchangers and accessory subunits) identified three genes encoding potassium channels associated with migraine, namely KCNK18, KCNG4 and KCNAB3 [100, 101].

(2) Vascular genes: These associated genes (ACE, MTHFR, NOTCH3, EDNRA) are involved in blood pressure regulation, endothelial cell function, vasoconstriction and vasodilation. Many vascular genes associated with migraine also confer risk for stroke and heart disease. These functional variants in some of vascular genes may cause migraine. Angiotensin converting enzyme (ACE) plays a key role in the maintenance of blood pressure and vessel wall tension. The D-D ("deletion-deletion") common variant located in the ACE gene (human chr. 17q23) increases ACE enzymatic activity, as well as the frequency and duration of MA attacks. MTHFR is a key component of the remethylation of homocysteine to methionine, as it catalyzes the conversion of 5,10-methylenetetrahydrofolate to 5-methyltetrahydrofolate. Rare loss-of-function mutations in the MTHFR gene, located in human chromosome 1p36.22, can lead to hyperhomocysteinemia due to decreased enzyme activity [102–109].

NOTCH3 encodes for a transmembrane receptor regulating vascular development and differentiation during embryogenesis, as well as contributing to vascular integrity in adults. In addition to rare NOTCH3 mutations producing MA within the context of CADASIL, also common variants are significantly associated with migraine. Hence, NOTCH3 may play a broader role also in the pathogenesis of common migraine, well beyond rare forms associated with CADASIL. Endothelial genes assessed for association with migraine encode for endothelin-1 (EDN1), endothelin receptor type A and B (EDNRA and EDNRB), inducible NO synthase (NOS2), endothelial NO synthase (NOS3) and vascular endothelial growth factor (VEGF) [110–114].

(3) Hormonal genes: These group genes are related with estrogen and progesterone metabolism especially relating to menstrual migraine. However, results from studies of genetic association between these genes and migraine were published in the later study, three estrogen receptor 1 (ESR1) haplotypes were significantly associated with the disorder ($P < 0.05$ or 0.01). In addition to ESR1, six other hormonal genes have been investigated, estrogen receptor 2 (ESR2), progesterone receptor (PGR) androgen receptor (AR), follicle stimulating hormone receptor (FSHR), nuclear receptor interacting protein 1 (NRIP1) and cytochrome P450, family 19, subfamily A, polypeptide 1 (CYP19A1) [115–119].

(4) Inflammatory genes: Recent studies shown that neurogenic inflammation, with activation of mast cells and macrophages accompanied by the release of proinflammatory cytokines may play an important role in the pathogenesis of migraine. Especially tumor necrosis factor alfa (TNF-α) gene variants is positive associated with migraine [120, 121]

4.2. Family linkage studies and GWAS

Many GWAS and classical linkage studies have been performed for migraine either using a genome-wide approach or targeting specific regions using microsatellite markers. Also, mitochondrial dysfunction in migraine that increased influx of calcium increases oxidative stress, that muscle biopsy of patients with migraine may show mitochondrial abnormalities, that mtDNA polymorphisms may be increased in migraine patients and that riboflavin, coenzyme-Q, niacin and carnitine, all agents used in the treatment of MIDs, exhibit a beneficial effect for migraine [122].

Recent GWAS studies have shown four SNPs, located on chromosome 8q22.1, 2q37.1, 12q13.3 and 1p36.32, which are associated with MA and/or MO. Although, some meta-analysis confirmed that the same results in independent populations. In another recent GWAS, three additional SNPs located at 1q22 and 3p24. However, all of these associated studies shown that the moderate of change in risk for migraine. On the other hand, the pedigree-based GWAS in an isolated population of Norfolk Island with a high prevalence of migraine and several novel variants in migraine susceptibility were identified [117–120].

4.3. Epigenetic

Epigenetics role of many complex diseases including migraine has aroused curiosity.

The effect of methylated DNA, methylated cytosines in the human D-loop of mitochondrial DNA (mtDNA), acetylation have shown differences between healthy controls and neurodegenerative and age-related diseases. Given comorbidities with migraine and the suggestive link between mitochondrial dysfunction and the lowered threshold for triggering a migraine attack, mitochondrial methylation may be a new avenue to pursue. New epigenetic approach of to solve the complex background of neurological diseases are very important [121–124].

The success of migraine genetic investigations will largely rely upon their capacity on one hand to apply the methodological approaches most apt to respond to each specific experimental question on the other hand, on their capacity to integrate multiple levels of phenotypic, functional and genetic information, in accordance with the complexity of the disorder itself. Environmental factors, such as early and recent life events, hormones and inflammation, can indeed act upon a genetically vulnerable background to trigger the onset and determine the progression of the disease.

Author details

Tuba Gökdoğan* Edgünlü[1] and Sevim Karakas Çelik[2]

*Address all correspondence to: tedgunlu@gmail.com

1 Department of Medical Biology, Medical Faculty, Muğla Sıtkı Koçman University, Muğla, Turkey

2 Department of Molecular Biology and Genetics, Science Faculty, Bülent Ecevit University, Zonguldak, Turkey

References

[1] Launer LJ, Terwindt GM, Ferrari MD. The prevalence and characteristics of migraine in a population-based cohort: the GEM study. Neurology 1999; 53: 537–542.

[2] Ahmed F. Headache disorders: differentiating and managing the common subtypes. Br J Pain 2012 Aug; 6 (3): 124–32.

[3] Headache Classification Subcommittee of the International Headache Society. The International Classification of Headache Disorders: 2nd edition. Cephalalgia 2004; 24(1): 9–160.

[4] Abu-Arafeh, I. Chronic tension-type headache in children and adolescents. Cephalalgia 2001; 21(8): 830–836.

[5] Unalp A, Dirik E, Kurul S. Prevalence and clinical findings of migraine and tension-type headache in adolescents. Pediatr Int 2007; 49(6): 943–949.

[6] Alzoubi K, Mhaidat N, Azzam S, Khader Y, Salem S, Issaifan H, Haddadin R. Prevalence of migraine and tension-type headache among adults in Jordan. J Headache Pain 2009; 10(4): 265–760.

[7] Kondratieva N, Azimova J, Skorobogatykh K, Sergeev A, Naumova E, Kokaeva Z, Anuchina A, Rudko O, Tabeeva G, Klimov E. Biomarkers of migraine: part 1—genetic markers. J Neurol Sci 2016 Oct 15; 369: 63–76. doi: 10.1016/j.jns.2016.08.008.

[8] Cho SJ, Song TJ, Chu MK. Outcome of Chronic Daily Headache or Chronic Migraine. Curr Pain Headache Rep 2016 Jan; 20(1): 2. doi: 10.1007/s11916-015-0534-8.

[9] Benoliel R, Eliav E. Primary headache disorders. Dent Clin North Am 2013 Jul; 57(3): 513–39.

[10] Russell MB. Genetics in primary headaches. J Headache Pain 2007 Jun; 8(3): 190–5.

[11] Pinessi L, Rainero I, Rivoiro C, Rubino E, Gallone S. Genetics of cluster headache: an update. J Headache Pain 2005 Sep; 6(4): 234–6.

[12] Rudkjobing LA, Esserlind AL, Olesen J. Future possibilities in migraine genetics. J Headache Pain 2012 Oct; 13(7): 505–11.

[13] Headache Classification Committee of the International Headache Society (IHS). The International Classification of Headache Disorders (3rd Edition). Cephalalgia 2013; 33(9): 629–808.

[14] Lyngberg AC, Rasmussen BK, Jørgensen T, Jensen R. Has the prevalence of migraine and tension-type headache changed over a 12-year period? A Danish population survey. Eur J Epidemiol 2005; 20(3): 243–9.

[15] Andlin-Sobocki P, Jönsson B, Wittchen HU, Olesen J. Cost of disorders of the brain in Europe. Eur J Neurol 2005 Jun; 12(1): 1–27.

[16] Schwartz BS, Stewart WF, Simon D, Lipton RB. Epidemiology of tension-type headache. JAMA 1998; 279: 381–383.

[17] Russell MB, Saltyte-Benth J, Levi N. Are infrequent episodic, frequent episodic and chronic tension-type headache inherited? A population-based study of 11 199 twin pairs. J Headache Pain 2006 Jun; 7(3): 119–26.

[18] Ulrich V, Gervil M, Olesen J. The relative influence of environment and genes in episodic tension-type headache. Neurology 2004 ; 62(11): 2065–9.

[19] Ostergaard S, Russell MB, Bendtsen L, Olesen J. Comparison of first degree relatives and spouses of people with chronic tension headache. BMJ 1997 Apr 12; 314(7087): 1092–3.

[20] Russell MB, Iselius L, Ostergaard S, Olesen J. Inheritance of chronic tension-type headache investigated by complex segregation analysis. Hum Genet 1998 Feb; 102(2): 138–40.

[21] Edgnülü TG, Özge A, Erdal N, Kuru O, Erdal ME. Association analysis of the functional MAOA gene promoter and MAOB gene intron 13 polymorphisms in tension type headache patients. Adv Clin Exp Med 2014 Nov-Dec; 23(6): 901–6.

[22] Männistö PT, Kaakkola S. Catechol-O-methyltransferase (COMT): biochemistry, molecular biology, pharmacology and clinical efficacy of the new selective COMT inhibitors. Pharmacol Rev 1999 Dec; 51(4): 593–628.

[23] Syvänen AC, Tilgmann C, Rinne J, Ulmanen I. Genetic polymorphism of catechol-O-methyltransferase (COMT): correlation of genotype with individual variation of S-COMT activity and comparison of the allele frequencies in the normal population and parkinsonian patients in Finland. Pharmacogenetics 1997 Feb; 7(1): 65–71.

[24] Zubieta JK, Heitzeg MM, Smith YR, Bueller JA, Xu K, Xu Y, Koeppe RA, Stohler CS, Goldman D. COMT val158met genotype affects mu-opioid neurotransmitter responses to a pain stressor. Science 2003 Feb 21; 299(5610): 1240–3.

[25] Fernández-de-las-Peñas C, Ambite-Quesada S, Rivas-Martínez I, Ortega-Santiago R, de-la-Llave-Rincón AI, Fernández-Mayoralas DM, Pareja JA. Genetic contribution of catechol-O-methyltransferase polymorphism (Val158Met) in children with chronic tension-type headache. Pediatr Res 2011 Oct; 70(4): 395–9.

[26] Ashina M. Neurobiology of chronic tension-type headache. Cephalalgia 2004 Mar; 24(3): 161–72.

[27] Colton CA, Brown CM, Cook D, Needham LK, Xu Q, Czapiga M, Saunders AM, Schmechel DE, Rasheed K, Vitek MP. APOE and the regulation of microglial nitric oxide production: a link between genetic risk and oxidative stress. Neurobiol Aging 2002 Sep-Oct; 23(5): 777–85.

[28] Gupta R, Kumar V, Luthra K, Banerjee B, Bhatia MS. Polymorphism in apolipoprotein E among migraineurs and tension-type headache subjects. J Headache Pain 2009 Apr; 10(2): 115–20.

[29] Banzi R, Cusi C, Randazzo C, Sterzi R, Tedesco D, Moja L. Selective serotonin reuptake inhibitors (SSRIs) and serotonin-norepinephrine reuptake inhibitors (SNRIs) for the prevention of tension-type headache in adults. Cochrane Database Syst Rev 2015 May 1; 5: CD011681.

[30] Gelernter J, Kranzler H, Coccaro EF, Siever LJ, New AS. Serotonin transporter protein gene polymorphism and personality measures in African American and European American subjects. Am J Psychiatry 1998; 155: 1332–8.

[31] Serretti A, Catalano M, Smeraldi E. Serotonin transporter gene is not associated with symptomatology of schizophrenia. Schizophr Res 1994; 35: 33–9.

[32] Mortensen OV, Thomassen M, Larsen MB, Whittemore SR, Wiborg O. Functional analysis of a novel human serotonin transporter gene promoter in immortalized raphe cells. Brain Res Mol Brain Res. 1999 May 7; 68(1–2): 141–8.

[33] Aylin A, Cengiz T, Emin E, Neriman A, Sacide P. Serotonin transporter gene polymorphisms in patients with chronic tension-type headache: a preliminary study. Neurol India 2008 Apr-Jun; 56(2): 156–60.

[34] Park JW, Kim JS, Kim YI, Lee KS. Serotonergic activity contributes to analgesic overuse in chronic tension-type headache. Headache. 2005 Oct; 45(9): 1229–35.

[35] Park JW, Kim JS, Lee HK, Kim YI, Lee KS. Serotonin transporter polymorphism and harm avoidance personality in chronic tension-type headache. Headache 2004 Nov-Dec; 44(10): 1005–9.

[36] Kusumi M, Araki H, Ijiri T, Kowa H, Adachi Y, Takeshima T, Sakai F, Nakashima K. Serotonin 2C receptor gene Cys23Ser polymorphism: a candidate genetic risk factor of migraine with aura in Japanese population. Acta Neurol Scand 2004 Jun; 109(6): 407–9.

[37] Frosst P, Blom HJ, Milos R, Goyette P, Sheppard CA, Matthews RG, Boers GJ, den Heijer M, Kluijtmans LA, van den Heuvel LP, et al. A candidate genetic risk factor for vascular disease: a common mutation in methylenetetrahydrofolate reductase. Nat Genet 1995 May; 10(1): 111–3.

[38] Kara I, Sazci A, Ergul E, Kaya G, Kilic G. Brain association of the C677T and A1298C polymorphisms in the 5, 10 methylenetetrahydrofolate reductase gene in patients with migraine risk. Res Mol Brain Res 2003 Mar 17; 111(1–2): 84–90.

[39] Kowa H, Yasui K, Takeshima T, Urakami K, Sakai F, Nakashima K. The homozygous C677T mutation in the methylenetetrahydrofolate reductase gene is a genetic risk factor for migraine. Am J Med Genet 2000 Dec 4; 96(6): 762–4.

[40] Ghosh J, Joshi G, Pradhan S, Mittal B. Investigation of TNFA 308G> A and TNFB 252G> A polymorphisms in genetic susceptibility to migraine. J Neurol 2010 Jun; 257(6): 898–904.

[41] Ghosh J, Pradhan S, Mittal B. Role of dopaminergic gene polymorphisms (DBH 19 bp indel and DRD2 Nco I) in geneticsusceptibility to migraine in North Indian population. Pain Med 2011 Jul; 12(7): 1109–11.

[42] Kusumi M, Ishizaki K, Kowa H, Adachi Y, Takeshima T, Sakai F, Nakashima K. Glutathione S-transferase polymorphisms: susceptibility to migraine without aura. Eur Neurol 2003; 49(4): 218–22.

[43] Tonon C, Guttmann S, Volpini M, Naccarato S, Cortelli P, D'Alessandro R. Prevalence and incidence of cluster headache in the Republic of San Marino. Neurology 2002; 58:1407–1409.

[44] Manzoni GC. Male preponderance of cluster headache is progressively decreasing over the years. Headache 1997; 37: 588–589.

[45] Russell MB. Epidemiology and genetics of cluster headache. Lancet Neurol 2004; 3: 279–283.

[46] Sjaastad O, Salvesen R. Cluster headache: are we only seeing the tip of the iceberg? Cephalalgia 1986; 6: 127–29.

[47] Sjaastad O, Shen JM, Stovner LJ, Elsas T. Cluster headache in identical twins. Headache 1993; 33: 214–17.

[48] Eadie MJ, Sutherland JM. Migrainous neuralgia. Med J Aust 1966; 1: 1053–57.

[49] Couturier EG, Hering R, Steiner TJ. The first report of cluster headache in identical twins. Neurology 1991; 41: 761–33.

[50] Roberge C, Bouchard JP, Simard D, Gagne R. Cluster headache in twins. Neurology 1992; 42: 1255–56.

[51] Svensson D, Ekbom K, Pedersen NL, Träff H, Waldenlind E. A note on cluster headache in a population-based twin register. Cephalalgia. 2003 Jun; 23(5): 376–80.

[52] Russell MB, Andersson PG, Thomsen LL. Familial occurrence of cluster headache. J Neurol Neurosurg Psychiatry 1995; 58(4): 341–343.

[53] Leone M, Russell MB, Rigamonti A, et al. Increased familial risk of cluster headache. Neurology 2001; 56(5): 1233–1236.

[54] El Amrani M, Ducros A, Boulan P, et al. Familial cluster headache: a series of 186 index patients. Headache 2002; 42: 974–977.

[55] De Simone R, Fiorillo C, Bonuso S, Castaldo G. A cluster headache family with possible autosomal recessive inheritance. Neurology 2003 Aug 26; 61(4): 578–9.

[56] Russell MB, Andersson PG, Thomsen LL, Iselius LJ. Cluster headache is an autosomal dominantly inherited disorder in some families: a complex segregation analysis. Med Genet 1995 Dec; 32(12): 954–6.

[57] Sjöstrand C, Russell MB, Ekbom K, Hillert J, Waldenlind E. Familial cluster headache. Is atypical cluster headache in family members part of the clinical spectrum? Cephalalgia 2005 Nov; 25(11): 1068–77.

[58] Shimomura T, Kitano A, Marukawa H, et al. Point mutation in platelet mitochondrial tRNA (Leu (UUR)) in patient with cluster headache. Lancet 1994; 27: 625–626.

[59] Cortelli P, Zacchini A, Barboni P, et al. Lack of association between mitochondrial tRNA (Leu(UUR)) point mutation and cluster headache. Lancet 1995; 345: 1120–1121.

[60] Seibel P, Grunewald T, Gundolla A, et al. Investigation on the mitochondrial transfer RNA(Leu)(UUR) in blood cells from patients with cluster headache. J Neurol 1996; 243: 305–307.

[61] May A, Bahra A, Buchel C, Frackowiak RS, Goadsby PJ. Hypothalamic activation in cluster headache attacks. Lancet 1998; 352: 275–278.

[62] Sakurai T, Amemiya A, Ishii M, et al. Orexins and orexin receptors: a family of hypothalamic neuropeptides and G protein-coupled receptors that regulate feeding behavior. Cell 1998; 92: 573–585.

[63] Nishino S. The hypocretin/orexin system in health and disease. Biol Psychiatry 2003; 54: 87–95.

[64] Siegel JM. Hypocretin (orexin): role in normal behavior and neuropathology. Annu Rev Psychol 2004; 55: 125–148.

[65] Dodick DW, Rozen TD, Goadsby PJ, Silberstein SD. Cluster headache. Cephalalgia 2000; 20: 787–803.

[66] De Lecea L, Kilduff TS, Peyron C, et al. The hypocretins: hypothalamus-specific peptides with neuroexcitatory activity. Proc Natl Acad Sci USA 1998; 95: 322–327.

[67] Rainero I, Gallone S, Valfrè W, et al. A polymorphism of the hypocretin receptor 2 gene is associated with cluster headache. Neurology 2004; 63: 1286–1288.

[68] Schurks M, Kurth T, Geissler I, Tessmann G, Diener HC, Rosskopf D. Cluster headache is associated with the G1246A polymorphism in the hypocretin receptor 2 gene. Neurology 2006; 66: 1917–1919.

[69] Rainero I, Gallone S, Rubino E, Ponzo P, Valfre W, Binello E, Fenoglio P, Gentile S, Anoaica M, Gasparini M, Pinessi L. Haplotype analysis confirms the association between the HCRTR2 gene and cluster headache. Headache 2008 Jul; 48(7): 1108–14.

[70] Baumber L, Sjostrand C, Leone M, et al. A genome-wide scan and HCRTR2 candidate gene analysis in a European cluster headache cohort. Neurology 2006; 66: 1888–1893.

[71] Rainero I, Rubino E, Valfrè W, Gallone S, De Martino P, Zampella E, Pinessi L. Association between the G1246A polymorphism of the hypocretin receptor 2 gene and cluster headache: a meta-analysis. J Headache Pain 2007 Jun; 8(3): 152–6.

[72] Weller CM, Wilbrink LA, Houwing-Duistermaat JJ, Koelewijn SC, Vijfhuizen LS, Haan J, Ferrari MD, Terwindt GM, van den Maagdenberg AM, de Vries B. Cluster headache and the hypocretin receptor 2 reconsidered: a genetic association study and meta-analysis. Cephalalgia 2015 Aug; 35(9): 741–7.

[73] Ofte HK, Tronvik E, Alstadhaug KB. Lack of association between cluster headache and PER3 clock gene polymorphism. J Headache Pain 2015 Dec; 17(1): 18.

[74] Katzenberg D, Young T, Finn T, Lin L, King DP, Takahashi JS, Mignot E. A Clock polymorphism associated with human diurnal preference. Sleep 1998; 21: 569–576.

[75] Cevoli S, Mochi M, Pierangeli G, Zanigni S, Grimaldi D, Bonavina G, Torelli P, Manzoni GC, Cortelli P, Montagna P. Investigation of the T3111C CLOCK gene polymorphism in cluster headache. J Neurol 2008 Feb; 255(2): 299–300.

[76] Rainero I, Rivoiro C, Gallone S, Valfrè W, Ferrero M, Angilella G, Rubino E, De Martino P, Savi L, Lo Giudice R, Pinessi L. Lack of association between the 3092 T→C Clock gene polymorphism and cluster headache. Cephalalgia 2005 Nov; 25(11): 1078–81.

[77] Welch KM, Nagesh V, Aurora SK, Gelman N. Periaqueductal gray matter dysfunction in migraine: cause or the burden of illness? Headache 2001; 41: 629–637.

[78] Rainero I, Rivoiro C, Rubino E, Milli V, Valfrè W, De Martino P, Lo Giudice R, Angilella G, Savi L, Gallone S, Pinessi L. Prevalence of HFE (hemochromatosis) gene mutations in patients with cluster headache. Headache 2005 Oct; 45(9): 1219–23.

[79] Olesen J, Thomsen LL, Lassen LH, Olesen IJ. The nitric oxide hypothesis of migraine and other vascular headaches. Cephalalgia 1995; 15: 94–100.

[80] Olesen J, Thomsen LL, Iversen H. Nitric oxide is a key molecule in migraine and other vascular headaches. Trends Pharmacol Sci 1994; 15: 149–53.

[81] Sjöstrand C, Modin H, Masterman T, Ekbom K, Waldenlind E, Hillert J. Analysis of nitric oxide synthase genes in cluster headache. Cephalalgia 2002 Nov; 22(9): 758–64.

[82] Rubino E, Ferrero M, Rainero I, Binello E,Vaula G, Pinessi L. Association of the C677T polymorphism in the MTHFR gene with migraine: a meta-analysis. Cephalalgia 2009; 29: 818–825.

[83] Schürks M, Rist PM, Kurth T. MTHFR 677C>T and ACE D/I polymorphisms in migraine: a systematic review and meta-analysis. Headache 2010; 50: 588–599.

[84] Goadsby PJ, Akerman S, Storer RJ. Evidence for postjunctional serotonin (5-HT1) receptors in the trigeminocervical complex. Ann Neurol 2001; 50: 804–807.

[85] Schürks M, Neumann FA, Kessler C, Diener HC, Kroemer HK, Kurth T, Völzke H, Rosskopf D. MTHFR 677C→T polymorphism and cluster headache. Headache 2011 Feb; 51(2): 201–7.

[86] Rainero I, Rubino E, Gallone S, Fenoglio P, Negro E, De Martino P, Savi L, Pinessi L. Cluster headache is associated with the alcohol dehydrogenase 4 (ADH4) gene. Headache 2010 Jan; 50(1): 92–8.

[87] Fourier C, Ran C, Steinberg A, Sjöstrand C, Waldenlind E, Belin CA. Screening of two ADH4 variations in a swedish cluster headache case-control material. Headache 2016 Apr 4.

[88] Siffert, W, et al. Association of a human G-protein b3 subunit variant with hypertension. Nat Genet 1998; 18: 45–48.

[89] Schürks M, Kurth T, Stude P, Rimmbach C, de Jesus J, Jonjic M, Diener HC, Rosskopf D. G protein beta3 polymorphism and triptan response in cluster headache. Clin Pharmacol Ther 2007 Oct; 82(4): 396–401.

[90] Sjöstrand C, Giedratis V, Ekbom K, Waldenlind E, Hillert J. CACNA1A gene polymorphisms in cluster headache. Cephalalgia 2001 Dec; 21(10): 953–8.

[91] Haan J, van Vliet JA, Kors EE, Terwindt GM, Vermeulen FL, van den Maagdenberg AM, Frants RR, Ferrari MD. No involvement of the calcium channel gene (CACNA1A) in a family with cluster headache. Cephalalgia 2001 Dec; 21(10): 959–62.

[92] Gasparini CF, Smith RA, Griffiths LR. Genetic insights into migraine and glutamate: a protagonist driving the headache. J Neurol Sci 2016 Aug 15; 367: 258–68.

[93] Russel MB, Iselius L, Olesen J. Migraine without aura and migraine with aura are inherited disorders. Cephalalgia 1996; 16: 305–309.

[94] Friedman DI, De ver Dye T. Migraine and the environment. Headache 2009; 49: 941–952.

[95] Nyholt DR, van den Maagdenberg AM. Genome-wide association studies in migraine: current state and route to follow. Curr Opin Neurol 2016 Jun; 29(3): 302–8.

[96] Federico A, Di Donato I, Bianchi S et al. Hereditary cerebral small vessel diseases: a review. J Neurol Sci 2012; 322: 25–30.

[97] Ophoff RA, DeYoung J, Service SK et al. Hereditary vascular retinopathy, cerebroretinal vasculopathy and hereditary endotheliopathy with retinopathy, nephropathy and stroke map to a single locus on chromosome 3p21.1-p21.3. Am J Hum Genet 2001; 69:447–453.

[98] Bersano A, Debette S, Zanier ER, et al. The genetics of smallvessel disease. Curr Med Chem 2012; 19: 4124–4141.

[99] Storimans CW, Van Schooneveld MJ, Oosterhuis JA, Bos PJ. A new autosomal dominant vascular retinopathy syndrome. Eur J Ophthalmol 1991; 1: 73–78.

[100] Terwindt GM, Haan J, Ophoff RA, et al. Clinical and genetic analysis of a large Dutch family with autosomal dominant vascular retinopathy, migraine and Raynaud's phenomenon. Brain 1998; 121(Pt 2): 303–316.

[101] Jen J, Cohen AH, Yue Q, et al. Hereditary endotheliopathy with retinopathy, nephropathy and stroke (HERNS). Neurology 1997; 49: 1322–1330.

[102] Vilotti S, Vana N, Van den Maagdenberg AM, Nistri A. Expression and function of calcitonin gene-related peptide (CGRP) receptors in trigeminal ganglia of R192Q Cacna1a knock-in mice. Neurosci Lett 2016 May 4; 620: 104–10. doi: 10.1016/j.neulet.2016.03.046. Epub 2016 Mar 25.

[103] Bürk K, Kaiser FJ, Tennstedt S, Schöls L, Kreuz FR, Wieland T, Strom TM, Büttner T, Hollstein R, Braunholz D, Plaschke J, Gillessen-Kaesbach G, Zühlke C. A novel missense mutation in CACNA1A evaluated by in silico protein modeling is associated with non-episodic spinocerebellar ataxia with slow progression. Eur J Med Genet 2014 Apr; 57(5): 207–11.

[104] Paterna S, Di Pasquale P, Cottone C, et al. Migraine without aura and ACE-gene deletion polymorphism: is there a correlation? Preliminary findings. Cardiovasc Drugs Ther 1997; 11: 603–604.

[105] Kowa H, Fusayasu E, Ijiri T, et al. Association of the insertion/deletion polymorphism of the angiotensin I-converting enzyme gene in patients of migraine with aura. Neurosci Lett 2005; 374: 129–131.

[106] Joshi G, Pradhan S, Mittal B. Role of the ACE ID and MTHFR C677T polymorphisms in genetic susceptibility of migraine in a north Indian population. J Neurol Sci 2009; 277: 133–137.

[107] Oterino A, Valle N, Bravo Y, et al. MTHFR T677 homozygosis influences the presence of aura in migraineurs. Cephalalgia 2004; 24: 491–494.

[108] Lea RA, Ovcaric M, Sundholm J, et al. Genetic variants of angiotensin converting enzyme and methylenetetrahydrofolate reductase may act in combination to increase migraine susceptibility. Brain Res Mol Brain Res 2005; 136: 112–117.

[109] Samaan Z, Gaysina D, Cohen-Woods S, et al. Methylenetetrahydrofolate reductase gene variant (MTHFR C677T) and migraine: a case control study and meta-analysis. BMC Neurol 2011; 11: 66.

[110] An XK, Lu CX, Ma QL, et al. Association of MTHFR C677T polymorphism with susceptibility to migraine in the Chinese population. Neurosci Lett 2013; 549: 78–81.

[111] Menon S, Cox HC, Kuwahata M, et al. Association of a notch 3 gene polymorphism with migraine susceptibility. Cephalalgia 2010; 31: 264–270.

[112] Tikka-Klemola P, Kaunisto MA, Hamalainen E, et al. Genetic association study of endothelin-1 and its receptors EDNRA and EDNRB in migraine with aura. Cephalalgia 2009; 29: 1224–1231.

[113] Joshi G, Pradhan S, Mittal B. Vascular gene polymorphisms (EDNRA -231 G>A and APOE HhaI) and risk for migraine. DNA Cell Biol 2011; 30: 577–584.

[114] Lemos C, Neto JL, Pereira-Monteiro J, et al. A role for endothelin receptor type a in migraine without aura susceptibility? A study in portuguese patients. Eur J Neurol 2011; 18: 649–655.

[115] Tzourio C, El AmraniM, Poirier O, et al. Association between migraine and endothelin type a receptor (ETA -231 A/G) gene polymorphism. Neurology 2011; 56: 1273–1277.

[116] Colson N, Fernandez F, Griffiths L. Genetics of menstrual migraine: the molecular evidence. Curr Pain Headache Rep 2010;14: 389–395.

[117] Colson NJ, Lea RA, Quinlan S, et al. The estrogen receptor 1 G594A polymorphism is associated with migraine susceptibility in two independent case/control groups. Neurogenetics 2004; 5: 129–133.

[118] Oterino A, Pascual J, Ruiz de Alegria C, et al. Association of migraine and ESR1 G325C polymorphism. Neuroreport 2006; 17: 61–64.

[119] Oterino A, Toriello M, Cayón A, et al. Multilocus analyses reveal involvement of the ESR1, ESR2 and FSHR genes in migraine. Headache 2008; 48: 1438–1450.

[120] Joshi G, Pradhan S, Mittal B. Role of the oestrogen receptor (ESR1 PvuII and ESR1 325 C->G) and progesterone receptor (PROGINS) polymorphisms in genetic susceptibility to migraine in a North Indian population. Cephalalgia 2010; 30: 311–320.

[121] Rainero I, Grimaldi LM, Salani G, et al. Association between the tumor necrosis factor-alpha -308 G/A gene polymorphism and migraine. Neurology 2004; 62: 141–143.

[122] Mazaheri S, Hajilooi M, Rafiei A. The G-308A promoter variant of the tumor necrosis factor-alpha gene is associated with migraine without aura. J Neurol 2006; 253: 1589–1593.

[123] Anttila V, Stefansson H, Kallela M, International Headache Genetics Consortium, et al. Genome-wide association study of migraine implicates a common susceptibility variant on 8q22.1. Nat Genet 2010; 42: 869–873.

[124] Kang DC, Su ZZ, Sarkar D, et al. Cloning and characterization of HIV-1-inducible astrocyte elevated gene-1, AEG-1. Gene 2005; 353: 8–15.

Chapter 2

Children and Adolescents with Primary Tension-Type Headaches: Research and Practice Perspectives for Non-Pharmacological Interdisciplinary Headache Service

Birte Tornøe

Additional information is available at the end of the chapter

http://dx.doi.org/10.5772/64971

Abstract

Background: Children and adolescents with frequent and chronic primary headaches are, with a prevalence of 2–23% depending on diagnosis, age, sex and frequency, a global health concern. Research on non-pharmacological treatment outcomes is sparse. Headache service faces a challenge because possible sensitisation of pain pathways can affect outcomes leading to a delay in becoming symptom free or being cured.

Method: This chapter provides a narrative review of research containing suggestions for relevant focus areas for professionals who work with children and their parents in the process of self-care.

Conclusions: Research supports that increased pericranial tenderness in children with consistent primary tension-type headache is a consequence of activated pain pathways and relevant for clinical assessment. Tension patterns, posture, muscle balance and strength in the neck/shoulder region are areas of importance for minimising the triggering of input to the nociceptive system. Lifestyle factors such as sleep, nutrition, stress and tension regulation, posture and ergonomics, physical activity (PA) and exercise are a key part of non-pharmacological team service. Empowering patient education that provides children and adolescents with the knowledge and drive to persistently pursue healthy lifestyle changes is the basis for potentially successful outcomes in terms of ethical, cultural and educational issues.

Keywords: children, headache service, empowering patient education, stress and tension regulation, aerobic power

1. Introduction

Children and adolescents with frequent and chronic primary headaches are, with a prevalence of 2–23% depending on diagnosis, age, sex and frequency, a global health concern [1–4]. The age span is 3–18 years depending on the disorder. The main consequences of frequent headaches in children and adolescents are more frequent school absences; disturbed health-related quality of life (HRQOL) [5] and a risk of medication overuse [6].

An interdisciplinary specialist team is a relevant health care platform for the professional support to the families in the process of self-care and recovery. A specialist team is suggested to consist of neuro-paediatricians, nurses, physiotherapists, psychologist and possibly a social worker [7].

The diagnosis of the child's headache as a neurological disorder is the first important step in an interdisciplinary team service and is carried out based on the International Classification of Headache Disorders (ICHD-3-beta) [8]. The most frequent diagnoses for children are migraine with or without aura, tension-type headache (TTH) or a combination of both, such as mixed headaches. Girls present the highest prevalence for TTH [4], but there is conflicting evidence as to whether boys or girls predominantly have mixed headache [1, 9].

There is a consensus that the aetiology and relevant factors are multi-dimensional with dynamic interaction between genetic, hormonal, neural and muscular mechanisms but also psycho-social and environmental factors. Researchers agree that migraine and TTH are two different headache disorders [1], though some see it as a continuum [9]. They may, however, interact, which is why efforts concerning TTH might be beneficial for the child with both disorders. Frequent and chronic types of headache, which means they occur more than 10–15 days a month, present the greatest challenge.

Research on non-pharmacological treatment outcomes is sparse. Headache service faces a challenge because possible sensitisation of pain pathways can affect outcomes leading to a delay in becoming symptom free or being cured. It is therefore important to empower children, adolescents and their involved parents to persistently pursue healthy lifestyle strategies, which could lead to a long-lasting reduction of headache frequency and prevent disability.

A narrative review [10] approach is used in the following sections to describe and discuss relevant areas of interest supported by research that might lead to headache reduction in children suffering from primary TTH.

2. Research on hypersensitivity

Langemark and Olesen were the first to focus on pericranial tenderness in adults with TTH [11]. Forty individuals with TTH and 40 controls were palpated by a blinded observer for tenderness in 10 pericranial bilateral sites using a four-point scale called the Total Tenderness Score (TTS) (**Table 1**). Results indicated a significant difference in tenderness between the two groups. Bendtsen et al. [12] examined later the use of a palpometer, which allowed measurement of palpation pressure during palpation. The palpometer was a small instrument with an arbitrary scale connected to a pressure-sensitive plastic device attached to the finger used for palpation. The use of the palpometer was recommended for research. Using the same observer between palpations was recommended to keep the amount of pressure stable. The TTS system was validated with the use of the palpometer [13].

0 No visible reaction and denial of tenderness
1 No visible reaction but verbal report of discomfort or mild pain
2 Verbal report of painful tenderness, facial expression of discomfort or no reaction
3 Marked grimacing or withdrawal, verbal report of marked painful tenderness and pain

Table 1. Langemark and Olesen's four-point total tenderness score [11].

Further research by Bendtsen et al. [14] focused on pericranial tenderness measured by a palpometer and TTSs; and pressure pain thresholds and tolerance recorded by an electronic pressure algometer at the non-dominant second finger and at the temporalis muscle. Similar to earlier studies the results showed significantly increased pericranial tenderness of all-sites-pericranial myofascial tissue in adult patients with chronic TTH (CTTH) compared with healthy controls. The results showed a decrease in pressure pain thresholds and tolerance, but these results were considered debatable. Results also showed a shift to the left compared with healthy controls when examining the functions for pressure pain thresholds and tolerance versus pain on both sites. The results were interpreted as indicators of general hypersensitivity in patients with CTTH.

At the time, there were also parallel studies focusing on children with headaches. For example, Carlsson [15] examined 113 Swedish schoolchildren with frequent headaches compared with 109 headache-free controls. The children were examined by manual palpation of seven bilateral pericranial sites and TTS. Children with headache had significantly higher tenderness, and children with chronic headaches had significantly higher tenderness for all sites, except the frontalis muscles. The mean tenderness scores were significantly correlated with the frequency of chronic tension-type headache (CTTH).

Additional studies involving children were conducted. Tornoe et al. [16] examined pericranial tenderness in 41 girls 9–18 years of age with frequent episodic TTH (FETTH) and CTTH compared with 41 healthy controls by means of TTS. Results showed significantly higher tenderness scores for girls with headache in all sites. Results showed a significant positive correlation between headache frequency and tenderness.

Soee et al. examined 59 children 7–17 years of age with FETTH and CTTH compared with 57 healthy controls. Examinations were conducted by means of the TTS at seven pericranial myofascial sites and the use of the original palpometer. Children with headache had significantly increased tenderness in all sites. The sites with the highest level of tenderness in children with and without headache were the trapezius descendens and its occipital insertions. Further examinations were conducted by means of algometry of pressure pain thresholds at three pericranial sites and suprapressure pain thresholds [17]. Sensitivity showed no significant increase measured by pressure pain and suprapressure pain thresholds compared with controls. Results from factor analyses indicated an association between pericranial tenderness and the child's general level of pain processing.

	Adults			Children		
Pericranial sites/studies	**Langemark and Olesen (1987)**	**Bendtsen et al. (1994–1996)**	**Jensen et al. (1992–1998)**	**Carlsson (1996)**	**Soee et al. (2013)**	**Tornoe et al. (2011–2016)**
M. Frontalis	X	X	X	X	X	X
M. Pterygoideus Medialis	X					
M. Pterygoideus Lateralis	X		X			
Hamulus Pterygoideus			X			
M. Masseter	X	X	X	X	X	X
Processus Coronoideus Mandibulae	X	X	X			
M. Sternocleido-Mastoideus	X	X	X	X	X	X
M. Trapezius	X	X	X	X	X	X
M. Temporalis	X	X	X	X	X	X
Processus Mastoideus	X	X	X	X	X	X
Occipital Muscle Insertions	X	X	X	X	X	X
M. Orbicularis Oculi				X		X
M. Corrugator Supercilii				X		
M. Rectus Capitis Posterior Major			X			
M. Splenius			X			

Table 2. Bilateral pericranial sites originally used in research for total tenderness score in TTH.

In another study, Soee et al. [18] conducted algometry and pain scoring for five increasing pressure intensities at two pericranial sites, the trapezius descendens and temporalis, on the non-dominant side. Fifty-eight children with FETTH and CTTH and 57 healthy controls participated. The area under the curve for stimulus-response functions was analysed. Similar to the results for adults in Bendtsen's [14] study, the stimulus-response functions for pressure versus pain showed a shift to the left, indicating hypersensitivity, especially for the group of children with CTTH. Soee et al. concluded that the temporalis site was the most sensitive and that quantitative and qualitative changes in pain perception occurred on a continuum, with

FETTH representing an intermediate state between healthy individuals and CTTH. In addition, Fernández-de-las-Peñas et al. [19] found bilateral pressure hypersensitivity in a study using the temporalis, trapezius descendens and tibialis anterior muscles in 25 children 5–11 years of age with FETTH compared with 50 healthy controls.

In a randomised controlled intervention trial with specific strength training versus interdisciplinary counselling [20], headache frequency and duration declined significantly over the space of 22 weeks, but pericranial tenderness did not change significantly in a positive direction. These results indicate that generally increased pericranial tenderness and hypersensitivity might predict a delay in becoming symptom free or being cured.

In summary, in both adults and children with TTH research support the findings of altered pain perceptions with hypersensitivity probably due to changes in both periphery and central pain pathways. A continuum between the healthy children and the children with chronic headaches is seen with the FETTHs as intermediates. The TTS as a palpation test seems an applicable and non-invasive examination for children in the clinic. To picture hypersensitivity tenderness in all pericranial sites would be expected. There is a need for revalidation of the TTS with the use of a calibrated palpometer in order to avoid large test-retest variations as found by Tornoe et al. [21] There is also a need for more research in order to establish a cut-off value between normal and pathological levels of tenderness in children. **Table 2** presents the bilateral pericranial sites originally used in research for TTS.

3. Tension patterns and self-regulation

Other names for TTH were tension headache and muscle contraction headache. Throughout the decades, various hypotheses and findings about the underlying mechanisms have served as a guide to developing a solid, evidence-based approach. In addition to research on pericranial myofascial tenderness and hypersensitivity, examining tension patterns in pericranial muscles and how to regulate tension and stress have also been of interest. Surface electromyographic biofeedback (SEMG) and progressive relaxation training have been examined with success in children suffering from TTH, though large-scale randomised controlled trials are still needed.

Focusing on the frontalis muscles, Grazzi et al. [22] examined SEMG biofeedback in 10 children 12–15 years of age with TTH. The children participated twice a week for 12 sessions and were also encouraged to use daily relaxation techniques at home. The results indicated a significant decrease in EMG activity and headache intensity from the first to the last session. Bussone et al. [23] did a subsequent larger controlled study with follow-up to 12 months. Their results showed a significant reduction in headache parameters but not in tension levels. The site was frontalis, and the feedback was auditory. In a 3-year follow-up study [24], results likewise showed long-lasting improvements after EMG biofeedback relaxation training for children with TTH, with further gains over the course of 3 years. Other researchers have examined biofeedback and relaxation therapy in various forms and find SEMG frontalis biofeedback to be superior. Results showed a long-lasting, continuously increasing effect [25]. The continuous effect indicates that children learn how to use and integrate the relaxation techniques into their daily lives.

Hermann and Blanchard [26] reviewed studies evaluating interventions with biofeedback and relaxation for children and reached an overall positive conclusion. They discussed how to distinguish between the input from biofeedback and the use of relaxation techniques, a distinction Kröner-Herwig et al. also make [25]. The question of whether the positive outcomes relate to an alteration in mental stress, muscular activity or a combination of the two was discussed and is still relevant.

Evidence on repetitive recruitment of motor units followed by pain, possibly altered muscle activation patterns and muscular cellular dysfunctions in adults with computer work-related trapezius myalgia has also propelled headache research. Even though the trapezius descendens (the upper trapezius) has been shown to be the most tender myofascial pericranial site in children with TTH, little research has been done on SEMG biofeedback from the trapezius muscle. One study compared frontalis SEMG biofeedback with trapezius SEMG biofeedback and progressive relaxation therapy alone in adults [27]. The results suggested that trapezius SEMG biofeedback training might be more efficacious for CTTH with a significant effect above 50%.

Children under the age of 13, who have not yet fully developed the ability to reason abstractly, need age-appropriate learning situations. Tornoe et al. [28] evaluated a study involving computer-animated SEMG biofeedback by placing sensors on the trapezius descendens and by employing an age-appropriate form of progressive relaxation techniques. The children, 7–13 years of age, worked with visual and auditory computer-animated feedback from screens showing brief videos. Additionally, a bar graph gave the child a visible response each time a certain tension threshold was exceeded. The sensor placement on the trapezius muscles provided the children a feedback from posture, breathing, tension and heart rate. Furthermore, SEMG data were also recorded. Comparing the pre-and post-treatment means of root mean squares and median frequencies showed a minor non-significant reduction for nine children across a nine-session programme. The SEMG results showed a significant within-session ability to up and down regulate tension. The study results showed a statistically significant reduction in headache frequency.

Oral and written evaluations by the children indicate that they felt they were able to moderate feelings of stress, multiple thoughts and emotions experienced as negative or stressing. The children likewise managed to regulate the way these mental phenomena presented in the body as increased heart rates, hyperventilation and/or muscle tension. Achieving a sufficient level of self-regulation experience and expertise appeared to require 9–10 sessions. Recent studies examined the additional use of internet-based self-help programmes and supported the applicability of the internet for cognitive-behavioural interventions [29], although evidence on headache reduction is conflicting [30]. **Figure 1** presents learning aspects of self-regulation.

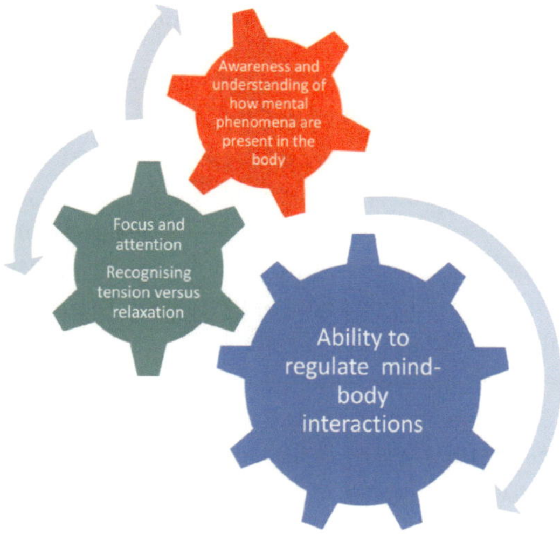

Figure 1. Using progressive relaxation techniques to learn self-regulation. This image belongs to the author of the chapter: PhD Birte Tornøe.

4. Lifestyle-related physical factors and resources

The neck/shoulder muscles are involved in the underlying pathology of headache. One hypothesis on adult patients with CTTH confirmed in findings was that higher tension levels measured by EMG in the trapezius muscles increase input from myofascial tissue leading to hypersensitivity [31]. Evidence of increased tension levels, however, shows conflicting results in adults, and EMG studies in children are sparse. A summary by Bendtsen and Fernandez-de-las-Penas [32] points out that prolonged nociceptive stimuli from myofascial input could be a result of continuous activation of local structures followed by microtrauma of selected muscle fibre, thus leading to increased hypersensitivity. They consequently recommended that specific attention be paid to the muscular factors underlying TTH [32]. From this perspective, the involvement of the trapezius muscles in computer-related workplace research is interesting. In a study involving adult females with trapezius myalgia, results from muscle biopsies indicated that women with trapezius myalgia had a higher percentage of hypertrophied type-I fibres with poor capillarisation. The findings were associated with long-term working exposure [33]. Recent studies on surface and intramuscular EMG support the involvement of subparts of the trapezius muscles related to both attention tasks and anticipatory motor programming of precise finger typing and manipulation. The latter could be approached with the use of elbow support, which would decrease the need for anticipatory shoulder stabilisation. Maintaining work-related local activity is believed to impair cellular mechanisms, leading to increased input to free nociceptive nerve endings [34]. In conclusion, both headache research and research in physiology and ergonomics support evidence on the involvement and impairment of subparts of the trapezius muscles in continuous daily, and especially work-related activities, leading to prolonged nociceptive input and hypersensitivity.

4.1. Posture, muscle activity and the use of electronic devices by children

Children and adolescents worldwide use iPads, computers and mobile phones for schoolwork and leisure activities. Children with TTH have been associated with more frequent use of computers than healthy controls [35]. Straker et al. [36] examined posture and muscle activity in young children with a mean age 5.6 years who were using either a tablet, desktop or paper. SEMG and 3-D-motion data were used to collect data. Desktop computers were associated with a more upright position and less muscle activity than both tablets and paper. On the other hand, desktop computers were associated with a more constrained and monotonous posture, while tablet and paper allowed for greater variation. The use of a tablet was associated with a more flexed posture, elevated shoulders and more muscular activity in the trapezius descendens muscles and cervical erector spinae. A study of children 10–12 years of age also indicated the same implications for computer use by children as are reported for adults. The mid position of the screen was shown to be the preferred position in terms of gaze, posture and muscle activity in the trapezius descendens and cervical erector spinae [37]. As a result, ergonomic advice and adjustments in the working environment for children with and without headache is recommended, particularly with the widespread use of tablets in schools and the amount of time spent using electronic devices. Straker et al. [38] reviewed the physical aspects of children's interaction with computers. The aim was to set up guidelines on how to use them wisely as a result of concerns about how extensive use of electronic devices might pose a risk to their development and health. A long list of recommendations emerged stressing that parents, teachers and health professionals have a responsibility to act and also to teach children how to use them prudently. Workplace adjustments, computer skills, body awareness (especially of bodily signals due to overload), transporting equipment, and physical exercise and activity are important to counter adverse consequences.

4.2. Muscle strength, aerobic power and health

In a historical review of research on physiology and ergonomics, Sjøgaard [39] shows that research indicates that physical exercise and activity can counteract the negative effects of muscular overload, producing a health-enhancing effect. Strength training in particular three times weekly for 10 weeks has a positive effect on muscular recovery. A study comprising girls 9–18 years of age with FETTH and CTTH found a significant association between headache and reduced neck/shoulder muscle strength and aerobic power [16]. Specific strength training of the trapezius descendens in particular was hypothesised to lead to significant headache reduction, which was confirmed in a later study [20]. At baseline the girls reported a perceived deficit in physical, emotional and school functioning domains and health measured by HRQOL questionnaires. Exercising and interdisciplinary counselling showed long-term improvements in these areas. Results indicated that the girls, who were interactive in exercising, gained greater physical results measured by strength and aerobic power than the girls who were verbally counselled to be more physically active.

The awareness of the importance of aerobic power in relation to headache is relatively new. The Norwegian HUNT3 study [40] also showed a significant inverse relationship between any type of headache and measured peak oxygen uptake in a sample of 3899 adults 20–50 years of age. Physical activity (PA) showed a similar relationship. It currently remains unclear as to what is cause and what is effect, but the truth is that perhaps they are both. Generally, muscular fitness, aerobic power (cardiorespiratory/cardiovascular fitness) and speed/agility are considered important markers for health in childhood [41], making this an important focus area for future research and interventions for children and adolescents with headache.

4.3. Sleep, nutrition and stress

Interdisciplinary counselling along with physical education for children and adolescents with TTH has a significant effect [20]. A recent study of 509 children 9–15 years of age with frequent weekly headaches [42] found that dysfunctional coping strategies for stress are negatively associated with the probability of headache remission. Other psychological variables were not significant. Girls presented higher prevalence and lower probability of remission than boys. Children, and especially girls, appear to need empowered learning on how to manage self-care in daily life by using active coping strategies. The perceived areas of deficit, such as physical, emotional and school functions, are of interest. Impaired school functioning is the least recognised area and needs further research. Examining and counselling on how to cope with and reduce stress and optimising sleep quality and nutrition are important areas to explore. An association has been confirmed between sleep difficulties and children with headache, which is why the underlying causes should also be addressed [43].

Enhancing PA is one way to regulate stress and to achieve better quality of sleep. The effect of PA on stress, anxiety, sleep quality and mental wellbeing may even be superior to mindfulness meditation and heart rate variability biofeedback [44, 45]. A certain amount of PA is necessary to maintain and improve aerobic power and health. Families should be empowered to follow the guidelines and recommendations set by the World Health Organization (WHO) [46]. **Figure 2** presents the possible interacting mechanisms underlying paediatric headache.

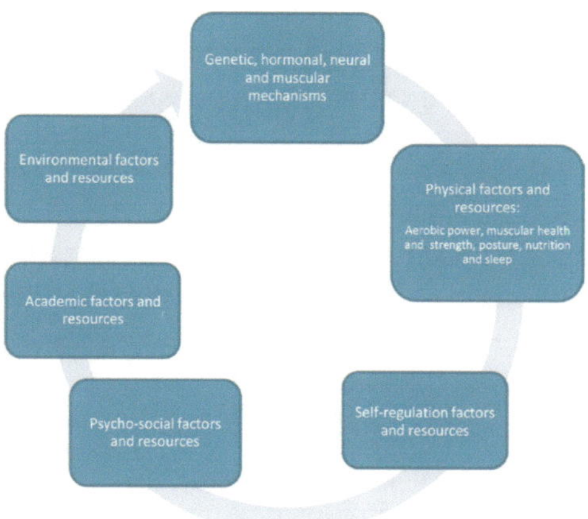

Figure 2. Possible interacting mechanisms underlying paediatric headache. This image belongs to the author of the chapter: PhD Birte Tornøe.

5. Empowering patient education

5.1. Empowerment

Over the years, health research has examined how to encourage the management of self-care in patients. Headache and other paediatric services face the challenge of how to empower the knowledge and understanding the children and parents have of specific focus areas and how to engage the child and parents in the process of changing health behaviour and incorporating active coping strategies.

The concept of empowerment developed in policy and social research in the 1960s and 1970s. From a medical perspective, Foucault stressed the need for patient knowledge, dialogue and shared decision-making [47]. Later, nursing research explored empowerment, with Leino-Kilpi defining the various dimensions of empowering patient education in a model to be used as a tool for examining and evaluating patient education [48]. The knowledge and skills acquired were the outcomes measured. Knowledge and knowledge expectations are key topics. A large European survey of adult surgical orthopaedic patients undergoing patient education concluded that knowledge and knowledge expectations differ between cultures and people depending on their background. The highest expectations were with regard to the bio-physiological and functional knowledge dimensions [49].

Aujoulat et al. [50] discussed the lack of conclusive definitions of empowerment but revealed a number of guiding principles. Empowerment is seen as both a process and an outcome [51, 52]. The empowerment process can be divided into two parts: (1) an intra-personal dimension where the individual transforms due to interactive learning and (2) an inter-personal dimension arising from the relationship between the patient and health provider [50, 51]. A key point is that an educational partnership is required to support and empower the patient (1) to collaborate, engage and be able to manage decision-making; (2) to gain knowledge and skills to cope with psycho-social and functional issues; (3) to have the right to self-determination; (4) to mobilise resources to become responsible and efficient in self-management; and (5) to adhere to mutual plans [48, 50, 53]. Time and experience are stressed as important factors in empowerment. Participation and interactive leaning are key topics [50, 51].

Child participation and decision-making are a specialist area as children are vulnerable participants in health care service. Decision-making involving children is linked to the ethical and legal rights of the child [54]. Children move through various stages of knowledge and cognitive skills, and have the right to participate regardless of the demands their developmental stage puts on how parents and professionals act. Generally, children develop their decision-making skills as they get older, with 18 the legal age of consent for treatment. Until then, professionals and parents act as proxies on behalf of the child and work in the child's best interest throughout childhood [55], even though children may not know their rights or may not want to participate. As a result, involved parents and professionals should encourage the child to participate and be interactive in learning and decision-making, but they should also respect the child's wishes and opinions [55]. Research points out that shared participation, decision-making and shared learning experiences with parents promote positive outcomes

http://dx.doi.org/10.5772/64971

[56], but in order to avoid an asymmetrical relationship, focusing on child-centred care, where the child is a key, active agent [57] guided by adults, is recommended.

As an advocate for adolescent-friendly health services, the WHO established quality standards in 2012 for this area [58], emphasising that services should be available, affordable and in an attractive environment. Ideally, adolescents should be involved in designing the service, which should provide up-to-date appropriate information and education that enables children and adolescents to make informed choices. Adolescents should be involved in monitoring and evaluating experiences. Interventions should be evidence-based, and the health service should encompass knowledge about general health needs. In addition, the health care staff should possess the necessary skills and be given sufficient time to provide care. Finally, all procedures should guarantee client confidentiality and value cultural and religious needs. In 2015, the European Health Parliament established a similar framework on patient empowerment and patient centredness [59].

5.2. How to facilitate health behaviour change

Various actors must be taken into consideration for health services, including the child, parents, professionals and the organisation, each of which perhaps has its own gender-specific culture and motivation. Research results show that additional fields of action must be examined in order to address these complex areas.

5.2.1. Child, parents and network

Engaging in PA decreases with age, though less so for boys than for girls [45, 60], indicating that this area needs more attention. In order to guide children to further pursue a physically active lifestyle, greater insight is needed into what key factors play a role. The Canadian Assessment of Physical Literacy (CAPL) [60] is an instrument validated in healthy children that offers assessment of PA, physical competence, motivation and confidence, knowledge and understanding related to a physically active lifestyle for children 8–12 years of age [60] and can provide insight into empowering elements. Further research will show whether CAPL can be used to benefit children with headache by pushing efforts in the right direction.

Little is known, in fact, about what motivates children. Trollvik et al. [61] examined what children experienced in a meaningful learning programme for children with asthma. The learning approach was varied and included storytelling, conversations, dialogue (including about bodily experiences) and interactive group activities. Qualitative evaluations based on recordings and observations showed that the following had a positive impact: (1) a warm and positive climate, (2) the opportunity to express and share feelings and reflections, (3) gaining new knowledge about the disorder and themselves and (4) interacting with other children and health care professionals. The study included a variety of communication methods to give the children both mental and bodily experiences.

Research indicates that parental participation plays an important role when children need empowering physical education [62]. Respecting the child/adolescent's needs, nurses and physical therapists can encourage and support families to make time to be physically active together, or to support the child, especially daughters, in other ways to promote a healthy lifestyle. Fathers and mothers influence their children differently, which is why health care staff should consider working with gender-specific approaches [63]. Parental support can be divided into actions that are instrumental, conditional, motivational and informational [63]. For example, parents can motivate their children and adolescents and give them information; and they can pay any expenses, for equipment and for transportation (instrumental). Direct parental involvement in PA (conditional), where the fathers' active involvement appears to be very important, is associated with increased levels of PA [45, 63]. Parental support has also been shown to result in the enhanced psycho-social wellbeing of the child [63]. Social support, including knowledge, beliefs and attitudes, from peers/friends and family also seem to have a clear positive effect on the PA level of adolescents [45, 63]. A positive climate, enjoyment and social elements are also known to facilitate the participation of children and adolescents [45], while a lack of time is perceived as a barrier [20, 45].

5.2.2. Professionals in the organisation

It is important to gain insight into the role, behaviour and thoughts of professional staff working in paediatric health care departments. Elwell et al. [64] conducted 33 interviews with clinical staff in inpatient and outpatient hospital services in order to identify the barriers and facilitators they experienced when providing advice to children and their families about healthy lifestyle behaviours. Barriers included a lack of time, a lack of feedback about whether the advice had had a positive impact and the constraints of working in a hospital environment. The facilitators included seeing health promotion as an important educational activity (not just information) that leads to cost savings, decreased admissions and better child health. In order to implement an educational activity that leads to positive outcomes, it is maintained that health care professionals must be trained. This argument is supported by Kelo et al. [56], who also examined how nurses perceive the utilisation of empowering education in school-aged children with diabetes and their parents. The study identified four phases or categories for successfully managing this process: assessment of knowledge, skills and needs, planning, implementation, including participation and interactivity, and finally evaluation and feedback for the family. It was stressed that educating children must be based on developmental psychology because of the various psychological and functional abilities that characterise the different ages [56, 65]. The study describes the complexity of an empowering patient education in detail, as well as the variety of approaches used. Nurses experienced management and leadership challenges due to a lack of expertise, a lack of resources and uncertainty. Also the situation of the child and parents, with their various attitudes and behaviours, was contained. The nurses experienced that, despite the challenges, empowering patient education made sense and contributed a positive learning effect for the participating children and their parents, which is an outcome that should be studied further.

The multiple components in this study clearly show that empowering patient education is a complex intervention that requires the organisation and professionals to adapt their work practices to accommodate the complexity [53, 56]. Homogenisation and standardisation in hospital organisations, however, may work to thwart the aim of empowering education and child centredness. **Figure 3** presents aspects of empowering patient education for children and adolescents with headache.

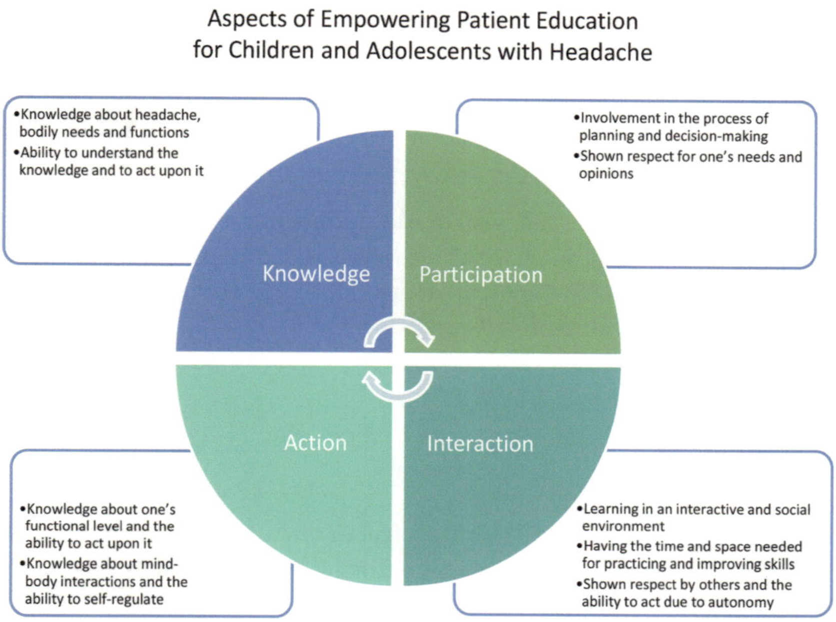

Figure 3. Aspects of empowering patient education for children and adolescents with headache. This image belongs to the author of the chapter: PhD Birte Tornøe.

6. Implications for headache service for children and adolescents

Empowering patient education has long-lasting positive outcomes for paediatric health care services. It implies giving the child, adolescent and involved parents a platform for experimental and interactive learning, where the child's right to autonomy and self-determination is respected and the child's motivation considered. Setting aside a sufficient amount of time is necessary for the various phases of a high-quality empowering educational programme, which include: examination, planning, education, implementation and, finally, evaluation and feedback. This involves managing a variety of communication and interactive methods. A child/adolescent-friendly atmosphere with pleasant social activities is empowering. These features combined mean that the staff who lead and manage the educational programmes must be prepared and have the necessary training. The organisation should also be able to encompass the complexity of the programme in order to live up to WHO and EU Health Parliament standards.

The educational content for children and adolescents with primary TTH is linked to general and specific health knowledge and skills. The strategies needed work to reduce psycho-physiological overload. Muscle load is seen leading to prolonged nociceptive input to pain pathways with subsequent hypersensitivity and chronic pain. Sufficient amounts of aerobic power achieved through training and outdoor play enhance health, and can also be used as active stress-coping strategies. Stress, sleep and nutrition hygiene also work to help accumulate the resources needed to cope with the demands of daily life and to reduce a psycho-physiological load.

Specific strength training, especially of the upper trapezius, might reverse negative muscular consequences from repetitive work with electronic devices. It is also necessary to reach a sufficient volume of training.

Relaxation training with SEMG and visual and auditory feedback is another interactive, effective learning process for children, which also tends to reduce prolonged nociceptive input. Awareness of and training on how to modulate workloads, posture, breathing and heart rate provides the knowledge and skills to self-regulate mind-body interactions in daily life.

7. Short conclusions

- Girls have a higher prevalence of TTH and a lower probability of headache remission, which is why children and adolescents may benefit from a headache service that focuses on the possibly different knowledge and needs of girls and boys.
- TTS is an applicable, non-invasive examination for children in the daily headache clinic. The palpation test can be used for examining pericranial tenderness as a consequence of pain hypersensitivity. Further research is needed to revalidate TTS with the use of a calibrated palpometer and to examine levels of sensitivity and specificity with cut-off values.
- Neck/shoulder muscles are involved in the underlying pathology of headache in children and adults. Muscle load from repetitive work can result in dysfunctions in muscular cellular mechanisms, thus leading to prolonged nociceptive input. Specific strength training, an adequate level of physical fitness and ergonomic learning can help restore the negative impact of repetitive work.
- Implementing relaxation techniques in paediatric educational programmes can also be beneficial. Courses must comprise at least ten sessions to provide the child and adolescent with enough time to experience how to work with and benefit from self-regulation techniques and stress-coping strategies, optionally combined with internet-based programmes. Computer-animated EMG biofeedback provides children with quick, easy and understandable visual and auditory feedback on the regulation of tension.
- Aerobic power is an important overall health marker for children and adolescents and is also a way to regulate stress. Parental participation and supportive behaviour play an important role in enhancing the PA of children, especially girls. A high level of PA also helps balance the time spent on electronic devices, which in turn has a positive impact on the child's health and development.

- Time and space to interact, practice and improve skills promotes successful outcomes for children and adolescents with headache. Shaping a social environment that involves interaction with friends and family is important to empower the child and adolescent to learn. A perceived lack of time, on the other hand, is a barrier in the daily life of families. More research is needed on how to approach this dilemma.
- The underlying mechanisms of headache are multi-systemic and involve various mental and physiological functions that need to be dealt with. Research indicates that the time span leading to successful outcomes lies between 3 months and 3 years. Setting aside time to develop and conduct high-quality, complex empowering educational programmes appears to raise the level of satisfaction and outcomes in children, adolescents, their involved parents and headache professionals.

Author details

Birte Tornøe

Address all correspondence to: birte.tornoee@gmail.com

1 Residence: Copenhagen, Denmark

2 Department of Health Sciences, Faculty of Medicine, Lund University, Sweden

References

[1] Waldie KE, Thompson JM, Mia Y *et al.* Risk factors for migraine and tension-type headache in 11 year old children. J Headache Pain 2014; 15:60.

[2] Gassmann J, Morris L, Heinrich M, Kroner-Herwig B. One-year course of paediatric headache in children and adolescents aged 8-15 years. Cephalalgia 2008; 28:1154–1162.

[3] Rho YI, Chung HJ, Lee KH *et al.* Prevalence and clinical characteristics of primary headaches among school children in South Korea: a nationwide survey. Headache 2012;52(4):592–599. DOI: 10.1111/j.1526-4610.2011.02001.x. Epub 2011 Sep 19.

[4] Zwart JA, Dyb G, Holmen TL *et al.* The prevalence of migraine and tension-type headaches among adolescents in Norway. The Nord-Trondelag Health Study (Head-HUNT-Youth), a large population-based epidemiological study. Cephalalgia 2004; 24:373–379.

[5] Strine TW, Okoro CA, McGuire LC, Balluz LS. The associations among childhood headaches, emotional and behavioral difficulties, and health care use. Pediatrics 2006; 117:1728–1735.

[6] Gelfand AA, Goadsby PJ. Medication overuse in children and adolescents. Curr Pain Headache Rep 2014; 18:428.

[7] Gaul C, Visscher CM, Bhola R *et al.* Team players against headache: multidisciplinary treatment of primary headaches and medication overuse headache. J Headache Pain 2011; 12:511–519.

[8] Headache Classification Committee of the International Headache Society I. The International Classification of Headache Disorders, 3rd edition (beta version). Cephalalgia 2013; 33:629–808.

[9] Genizi J, Khourieh Matar A, Schertz M *et al.* Pediatric mixed headache—The relationship between migraine, tension-type headache and learning disabilities—in a clinic-based sample. J Headache Pain 2016; 17:42.

[10] Green BN, Johnson CD, Adams A. Writing narrative literature reviews for peer-reviewed journals: secrets of the trade. J Sports Chiropr Rehabil 2001; 15:5–19.

[11] Langemark M, Olesen J. Pericranial tenderness in tension headache. A blind, controlled study. Cephalalgia 1987; 7:249–255.

[12] Bendtsen L, Jensen R, Jensen NK, Olesen J. Muscle palpation with controlled finger pressure: new equipment for the study of tender myofascial tissues. Pain 1994; 59:235–239.

[13] Bendtsen L, Jensen R, Jensen NK, Olesen J. Pressure-controlled palpation: a new technique which increases the reliability of manual palpation. Cephalalgia 1995; 15:205–210.

[14] Bendtsen L, Jensen R, Olesen J. Decreased pain detection and tolerance thresholds in chronic tension-type headache. Arch Neurol 1996; 53:373–376.

[15] Carlsson J. Tenderness of pericranial muscles in schoolchildren with headache. The Pain Clinic 1996; 9:49–56.

[16] Tornoe B, Andersen LL, Skotte JH *et al.* Reduced neck-shoulder muscle strength and aerobic power together with increased pericranial tenderness are associated with tension-type headache in girls: a case-control study. Cephalalgia 2013;34(7):540–547.

[17] Soee AB, Skov L, Kreiner S *et al.* Pain sensitivity and pericranial tenderness in children with tension-type headache: a controlled study. J Pain Res 2013; 6:425–434.

[18] Soee AB, Thomsen LL, Kreiner S *et al.* Altered pain perception in children with chronic tension-type headache: is this a sign of central sensitisation? Cephalalgia 2013; 33:454–462.

[19] Fernandez-de-Las-Penas C, Fernandez-Mayoralas DM, Ortega-Santiago R *et al.* Bilateral, wide-spread, mechanical pain sensitivity in children with frequent episodic tension-type headache suggesting impairment in central nociceptive processing. Cephalalgia 2010; 30:1049–1055.

[20] Tornoe B, Andersen LL, Skotte JH *et al.* Specific strength training compared with interdisciplinary counseling for girls with tension-type headache: a randomized controlled trial. J Pain Res 2016; 9:257–270.

[21] Tornoe B, Andersen LL, Skotte JH *et al.* Test-retest repeatability of strength capacity, aerobic power and pericranial tenderness of neck and shoulder muscles in children-relevant for tension-type headache. J Pain Res 2013; 6:1–9.

[22] Grazzi L, Leone M, Frediani F, Bussone G. A therapeutic alternative for tension headache in children: treatment and 1-year follow-up results. Biofeedback Self Regul 1990; 15:1–6.

[23] Bussone G, Grazzi L, D'Amico D *et al.* Biofeedback-assisted relaxation training for young adolescents with tension-type headache: a controlled study. Cephalalgia 1998; 18:463–467.

[24] Grazzi L, Andrasik F, D'Amico D *et al.* Electromyographic biofeedback-assisted relaxation training in juvenile episodic tension-type headache: clinical outcome at three-year follow-up. Cephalalgia 2001; 21:798–803.

[25] Kröner-Herwig B, Mohn U, Pothmann R. Comparison of biofeedback and relaxation in the treatment of pediatric headache and the influence of parent involvement on outcome. Appl Psychophysiol Biofeedback 1998; 23:143–157.

[26] Hermann C, Blanchard EB. Biofeedback in the treatment of headache and other childhood pain. Appl Psychophysiol Biofeedback 2002; 7:143–162.

[27] Arena JG, Bruno GM, Hannah SL, Meador KJ. A comparison of frontal electromyographic biofeedback training, trapezius electromyographic biofeedback training, and progressive muscle relaxation therapy in the treatment of tension headache. Headache 1995; 35:411–419.

[28] Tornoe B, Skov L. Computer Animated Relaxation Therapy in Children between 7 and 13 Years with Tension-Type Headache: A Pilot Study. Appl Psychophysiol Biofeedback 2012;37:35–44.

[29] Trautmann E, Kroner-Herwig B. A randomized controlled trial of Internet-based self-help training for recurrent headache in childhood and adolescence. Behav Res Ther 2010; 48:28–37.

[30] Law EF, Beals-Erickson SE, Noel M *et al.* Pilot randomized controlled trial of internet-delivered cognitive-behavioral treatment for pediatric headache. Headache 2015; 55:1410–1425.

[31] Jensen R, Bendtsen L, Olesen J. Muscular factors are of importance in tension-type headache. Headache 1998; 38:10–17.

[32] Bendtsen L, Fernandez-de-las-Penas C. The role of muscles in tension-type headache. Curr Pain Headache Rep 2011; 15:451–458.

[33] Andersen LL, Suetta C, Andersen JL *et al.* Increased proportion of megafibers in chronically painful muscles. Pain 2008; 139:588–593.

[34] Sogaard K, Olsen HB, Blangsted AK, Sjogaard G. Single motor unit firing behavior in the right trapezius muscle during rapid movement of right or left index finger. Front Hum Neurosci 2014; 8:881.

[35] Oksanen A, Metsahonkala L, Anttila P *et al.* Leisure activities in adolescents with headache. Acta Paediatr 2005; 94:609–615.

[36] Straker LM, Coleman J, Skoss R *et al.* A comparison of posture and muscle activity during tablet computer, desktop computer and paper use by young children. Ergonomics 2008; 51:540–555.

[37] Straker L, Burgess-Limerick R, Pollock C *et al.* Children's posture and muscle activity at different computer display heights and during paper information technology use. Hum Factors 2008; 50:49–61.

[38] Straker L, Maslen B, Burgess-Limerick R *et al.* Evidence-based guidelines for the wise use of computers by children: physical development guidelines. Ergonomics 2010; 53:458–477.

[39] Sjøgaard G. The August Krogh Institute: capillaries and beyond. Scand J Med Sci Sports 2015; 25(Suppl. 4):16–21.

[40] Hagen K, Wisloff U, Ellingsen O et al. Headache and peak oxygen uptake: The HUNT3 study. Cephalalgia 2016;36(5):437–444 DOI: 10.1177/0333102415597528. Epub 2015 Jul 23.

[41] Ortega FB, Ruiz JR, Castillo MJ, Sjostrom M. Physical fitness in childhood and adolescence: a powerful marker of health. Int J Obes (Lond) 2008; 32:1–11.

[42] Carasco M, Kroner-Herwig B. Psychological predictors of headache remission in children and adolescents. Adolesc Health Med Ther 2016; 7:59–66.

[43] Dosi C, Figura M, Ferri R, Bruni O. Sleep and headache. Semin Pediatr Neurol 2015; 22:105–112.

[44] van der Zwan JE, de Vente W, Huizink AC *et al.* Physical activity, mindfulness meditation, or heart rate variability biofeedback for stress reduction: a randomized controlled trial. Appl Psychophysiol Biofeedback 2015; 40:257–268.

[45] Biddle SJH, Mutrie N. Psychology of Physical Activity. Determinants, Well-Being and Interventions. 2nd ed. Taylor & Francis Group, New York: Routledge; 2010. p. 2–136.

[46] WHO. Global Recommendations on Physical Activity for Health. 2011. Available from: www.who.int/topics/physical_activity

[47] Foucault M. The Birth of the Clinic. Taylor & Francis Group, New York: Routledge; 2010. p. 1–25.

[48] Leino-Kilpi H, Luoto E, Katajisto J. Elements of empowerment and MS patients. J Neurosci Nurs 1998; 30:116–123.

[49] Valkeapaa K, Klemetti S, Cabrera E *et al.* Knowledge expectations of surgical orthopaedic patients: a European survey. Int J Nurs Pract 2014; 20:597–607.

[50] Aujoulat I, d'Hoore W, Deccache A. Patient empowerment in theory and practice: polysemy or cacophony? Patient Educ Couns 2007; 66:13–20.

[51] Cheryl H, Gibson CH. The process of empowerment in mothers of chronically ill children. J Adv Nurs 1995; 21:1201–1210.

[52] Rappaport J. Studies in Empowerment: Introduction to the Issue. Pennsylvania: Haworth Press; 1984. p. 1–7.

[53] Cheryl H, Gibson CH. A concept analysis of empowerment. J Adv Nurs 1991; 16:354–361.

[54] UN. Convention on the Rights of the Child. 1989. Available from: www.unicef.org/crc.

[55] Hallstrom I, Elander G. Decision making in paediatric care: an overview with reference to nursing care. Nurs Ethics 2005; 12:223–238.

[56] Kelo M, Eriksson E, Eriksson I. Pilot educational program to enhance empowering patient education of school-age children with diabetes. J Diabetes Metab Disord 2013; 12:16.

[57] Coyne I, Hallstrom I, Soderback M. Reframing the focus from a family-centred to a child-centred care approach for children's healthcare. J Child Health Care 2016; May 1. pii: 1367493516642744. [Epub ahead of print] DOI:10.1177/1367493516642744.

[58] WHO. Making Health Services Adolescent Friendly. Developing National Quality Standards for Adolescent Friendly Health Services. Geneva: WHO; 2012. Available from: www.who.int/maternal_child_adolescent/

[59] EU. Patient Empowerment and Centredness. 2015. Available from: www.healthparliament.eu.

[60] Longmuir PE, Boyer C, Lloyd M *et al.* The Canadian assessment of physical literacy: methods for children in grades 4 to 6 (8 to 12 years). BMC Public Health 2015; 15:767.

[61] Trollvik A, Ringsberg KC, Silen C. Children's experiences of a participation approach to asthma education. J Clin Nurs 2013; 22:996–1004.

[62] Lindqvist AK, Kostenius C, Gard G, Rutberg S. Parent participation plays an important part in promoting physical activity. Int J Qual Stud Health Well-being 2015; 10:27397.

[63] Beets MW, Cardinal BJ, Alderman BL. Parental social support and the physical activity-related behaviors of youth: a review. Health Educ Behav 2010; 37:621–644.

[64] Elwell L, Powell J, Wordsworth S, Cummins C. Health professional perspectives on lifestyle behaviour change in the paediatric hospital setting: a qualitative study. BMC Pediatr 2014; 14:71.

[65] Webber GC. Patient education. A review of the issues. Med Care 1990; 28:1089–1103.

Primary Headaches and their Relationship with the Autonomic Nervous System

Cuciureanu Dan Iulian, Constantinescu Irina,
Constantinescu Victor, Corciova Calin and
Matei Daniela

Additional information is available at the end of the chapter

http://dx.doi.org/10.5772/65737

Abstract

Headache disorders, described as early as 3000 BC, represent both a treatment challenge and a serious public health concern, with impact on the individual and society. Existing research in primary headache syndromes (not being caused by any underlying problem) focuses mainly on pain mechanisms. However, the painful symptomatology is the main encounter for the decreased quality of life and discomfort, the vegetative manifestations that frequently accompany the cephalalgic syndromes represent an important source of distress. Despite the advancement of the understanding of the molecular basis of headache disorders and neurovascular complex interactions, there is still lack of a cohesive understanding of the neurovegetative modulation in different types of primary cephalalgic syndromes. The aim of this chapter is to present an overview of the neurochemical mechanisms and pathways, which subtend dysautonomic manifestations in headache.

Keywords: headache, autonomic dysfunction, neurovascular system, heart rate variability, sympathetic nervous system

1. Introduction

The foundation of our current understanding of the mechanisms of headache dates back to seventeenth century, when Thomas Willis, one of the great figures in medicine, proposed that the source of pain was not the brain itself, but nerve fibers being pulled by the distended vessels. He therefore postulated the vascular theory of headache. It is known today that the autonomic manifestations of the vascular headaches are provoked by the tight connections between the pain receptors located at the head level and the autonomic structures of the central nervous system. The primary cephalalgic syndromes with vascular implications (migraine, cluster headache, SUNCT, and paroxysmal hemicrania) present intricate pathogenic mechanisms, involving autonomic centers of the brain stem. Therefore, headache's complex manifestations must be understood based on anatomical and physiological correlations with pain sensitive structures of the cranium.

Primary headaches define "idiopathic" types of cephalgia, which are not the result of an underlying disease or process. However, these conditions seem to be the result of a complex interaction among genetic, developmental, and environmental risk factors. The World Health Organisation (WHO) considers headache disorders as a major public-health concern, given the individual and social impact and financial costs to society [1]. Migraine—one of the most common primary headaches—is now ranked by the WHO as number 19 among all diseases worldwide causing disability.

During the last years, the classification of headaches has undergone a dynamic process of restructuration, more detailed specifications to each entity being gradually added, due to the advancement in the understanding of the pathophysiological mechanisms. The International Headache Society (IHS) classifies primary headaches into four main categories: migraine (with its subtypes), tension-type headache, cluster headache and other trigeminal autonomic cephalgias, and other primary headaches [2].

Migraine is characterized by attacks of moderate to severe unilateral and pulsatile headache lasting for 4–72 h, which is often associated with photophobia, phonophobia, nausea, and vomiting. In migraine with aura, the headache may be preceded by transient focal neurological symptoms. Trigeminal autonomic cephalalgias (TACs) are a group of primary headaches characterized by lateralized headache and ipsilateral cranial autonomic features such as conjunctive injection, lacrimation, and rhinorrhea. The main subtypes are represented by cluster headache, paroxysmal hemicrania, short-lasting unilateral neuralgiform headache attacks with conjunctival injection and tearing (SUNCT)/short-lasting unilateral neuralgiform headache attacks with cranial autonomic features (SUNA), and hemicrania continua [2]. The TACs are distinguished from each other by their attack length, duration, and frequency of occurrence [2].

Preclinical studies in primary headaches highlighted the complex and intricate mechanisms involving the anatomy and physiology of trigeminovascular and cranial autonomic systems responsible for a variety of symptoms [3–5]. The nociceptive innervation of intracranial vessels and the meninges is based on unmyelinated (C-fibers) and thinly myelinated (Aδ fibers) axons containing vasoactive neuropeptides such as substance P (SP) and calcitonin gene-related peptide (CGRP) [6]. Besides the trigeminal fibers originating in the ipsilateral trigeminal ganglion, neurovegetative fibers formed mainly by sympathetic tracts arising mainly from the superior cervical ganglion and a rather sparse innervation by parasympathetic fibers originating in the sphenopalatine and otic ganglia have been described [7, 8]. The innervation of intracerebral (pial) blood vessels has also an autonomic component, represented mainly by

http://dx.doi.org/10.5772/65737

parasympathetic fibers coming principally from the internal carotid and sphenopalatine ganglia [9].

However, despite an increasing body of data concerning the morphofunctional organization of the pain system in headache, the episodic and rather unpredictable manifestations of most primary headaches still represent a clinical and therapeutic challenge. There are numerous hypotheses at different levels, from molecular signaling to brain networks, with more and more data defining the "pain matrix" as a top-down system, implying both central and peripheral structures, from impairment in the functional connectivity during resting state (default mode network) to neurogenic inflammation mediating vasodilatation and increased permeability of blood vessels [10, 11].

2. Complex neurovascular interactions in primary headaches: migraine as a pathophysiological model

Primary headaches share many similarities, primarily trigeminovascular activation. While migraine is the most studied of all primary headaches, from both a clinical and a preclinical perspective, there have been advances in our understanding of the pathophysiology of tension-type headache and the trigeminal autonomic cephalalgias, through a combination of clinical studies and preclinical animal models.

Migraine is a complex primary brain disorder that involves a cascade of events that lead to recurrent inappropriate activations of the trigeminocervical pain system. As any other pain, it is perceived differently by each patient. Conceived as an alarm system of the body, the pain may become, at some point, an aggressor factor of the own body by the reflex reactions that it can trigger. It is well known that the pain perception is dependent not only on the intensity of the stimulus, but also on a multitude of genetic, psychological associated factors (emotional state and attention), on anterior experiences, memories, associations with facts of life, and comorbidities. The stimulation of the nociceptors in teguments, vessels, and joints leads the stimulus on known sensitive paths toward the parietal cortex, but a series of regulating neural mechanisms intervene both at the cortical level and on the route of the stimulus, trying to adapt the perception of the pain sensation to the individual body homeostasis. Which are those structures and whether they can be influenced represent the concern of scientists for decades.

The meningeal vessels have a motor and sensitive innervation by the trigeminal terminations (ophthalmic branches for the anterior and posterior compartment, the cervical C2, C3 nerve roots, with sympathetic fibers from the paravertebral sympathetic chain-contributing for the posterior part), which, in the end, establish connections with the secondary trigeminal neurons from the caudal trigeminal nucleus. Trigeminal nucleus is made up of the spinal portion in the converging information about pain and temperature and the pontine region with tactile information. The dendrites of the bipolar neurons from Gasser ganglia receive input from the pain receptors of dura mater and craniofacial structures, but also from the vascular wall and they direct it to trigeminal nucleus, thalamus, and contralateral parietal cortex (and in the same time collateral projections also target mesencephalic nuclei), including the dorsal reticular nucleus (DRt), the rostral ventral medulla (RVM), and the midbrain periaqueductal gray (PAG) [12–14].

The motor component of the cerebrovascular system implies an extrinsic innervation of the meningeal vessels, from the cervical (sympathetical), otic, sphenopalatin, and trigeminal ganglia (parasympathetical) and an intrinsic innervation for the small intraparenchimatous vessels, derived from brain stem nuclei such as locus coeruleus [15].

Cerebral blood flow (CBF) is regulated by vasomotor, chemical, metabolic, and neurogenic mechanisms, but under normal physiological conditions neurogenic control has little influence on cerebral autoregulation as other methods of control are dominant [16].

There is considerable experimental literature to document that stimulation of trigeminal afferents can result in cranial autonomic outflow, the trigeminal–autonomic reflex.

From the time of the stimulation of the nociceptive endings until the perception of the pain sensation, the transmission of the signal is modified by a series of mechanisms with the final aim of improving the painful sensation.

3. Nociceptive system modulation in primary headaches

Known in a great measure, the endogenous antinociceptive system is organized on three levels: first, supraspinal descending inhibition; second, segmental spinal inhibition (inhibitor complex of the pain in the posterior horn of the spine), and third, propriospinal, heterosegmental inhibition-supraspinal descending inhibition system.

The experimental studies, using pharmacological techniques, inhibitors, electrical stimulators, and functional neuroimaging techniques, revealed the existence of a complex system of pain modulation, a real neuronal matrix that is highly activated at the arrival of a nociceptive stimulus. This network is a dynamic and plastic connection between different neuronal relays and it is also involved in other higher nervous activities: cognition, emotion, and motivation. The pain network, with an anatomical basis still partially known, involves a series of neuromodulators and receptors and may be influenced both pharmacologically (including opiates, cannabinoids, NSAIDs, and serotonin/norepinephrine reuptake blockers) and mentally and emotionally, ultimately determining the sensation of pain [17].

Anatomically, the parietal cortex 1 and 2, insular lobe, thalamus, hypothalamus, amygdala, and the rostral anterior cingulate cortex (rACC) send messages to the periaqueductal gray matter (PAG) from where the descending inhibitor stimulus is transmitted to the trunk (sensory trigeminal core) and rostral bone marrow, with descending inhibitory projection on the medullar posterior horn.

The periaqueductal gray matter is a real center for holistic integration of the painful sensation because it has connections with the prefrontal cortex and amygdala, which, in turn, have a recognized role in the integration of emotions, anxiety, and risk assessment with avoidance [18].

Fields et al. [19] have identified in the rostral cervical region the existence of two neuronal populations with different functional roles: population "on" which increases its discharges before initiating the nociceptive reflex, and the population "off" which reduces its discharges when responding to the pain and whose activation produces analgesia. The population "on" is represented by the μ-opioid receptors whose activation inhibits the discharges of these neurons. Opioids and cannabinoids inhibit pain by enhancing the baseline firing rate of "off"-cells and eliminating the "off"-cells pause in response to nociceptive stimuli [20]. In these interdependent connections, a series of neuromediators may have multiple actions, such as serotonin and norepinephrine, but also other aminergic systems.

The PAG and RVM stimulation determine the release of serotonin, as the nucleus raphe magnus located near the trigeminal nucleus, in the bilateral inferior arch, releases serotonin with a possible role in the process of endogenous analgesia. The functional neuroimaging using BOLD technique revealed the activation of the nucleus as answer to the trigeminal painful stimulation suggesting its role [14, 21, 22].

Conversely, the implication of serotonin in stimulating the PAG and RVM neurons is not fully understood, but it is obvious that other nonserotonergic systems are involved in modulating the pain. Serotonin could be both inhibitory and facilitating the pain depending on the subtype of receptors excited. That GABAergic and glycinergic projections from the RVM mediate antinociception [23].

Norepinephrine released by the locus coeruleus and Kölliker-Füse nuclei under the impulses arrived from PAG and RVM seem to have a strong antinociceptive role by blocking the pre- and postsynaptic receptors of the spinal neurons involved in transmitting the pain or by stimulating the alpha-2-adrenergic receptors and indirectly by stimulating the alpha-1-receptors, which will cause the depolarization of inhibitory GABAergic neurons [23].

3.1. Segmental spinal inhibition

At the posterior horn of the spine, the endogenous antinociceptive system is represented by interneurons and the supramedullary descending endings. The opioids act on μ receptors located on the presynaptic endings of the related fibers where it blocks the calcium channels and open the potassium channels producing a hyperpolarization by inhibiting the release of neurotransmitter and thus analgesia. The endogenous analgesic system that is usually inactive and whose center is PAG projects from it axons (enkephalin conductors) to the raphe magnus nucleus, and from here to the interneurons from the posterior horn where they can secrete serotonin facilitating the release of enkephalins from the spinal interneurons. The interneurons receive external nociceptive fibers and the enkephalins from the two sources are blocking presynaptically the nociceptive signal. The stimulation of the opioid receptors from the related nociceptive fibers by enkephalin will determine the same blockage of the calcium channels whose activation is also necessary for releasing the substance P [24]. Supraspinal descending inhibition may not only depress mean discharge rates of nociceptive spinal dorsal horn neurons, but also may modify harmonic oscillations and nonlinear dynamics (dimensionality) of discharges [25].

3.2. Propriospinal, heterosegmental inhibition

Besides the classical, local, segmental, and supraspinal descending systems, it seems that there is a third endogenous antinociceptive system: propriospinal, intersegmental system inhibiting the nociceptive neurons in the dorsal horn. It seems to modulate partially the descending pathways and it is activated by conditioning (stimulating) the heterosegmental painful stimuli causing a neuronal constrastimulation (counterirritation) [25].

This multistage organization of the endogenous antinociceptive system can be influenced with beneficial results or it can be demodulated resulting in pain exacerbation.

The new functional neuroimaging techniques have showed the influence of the placebo-type psychogenic factor that cause the activation of the descending inhibitory network with the stimulation of the μ-opioids in rostral anterior cingulate cortex (rACC), the posterior cingulate cortex(PCC), the dorsolateral prefrontal cortex, and the anterior insular cortex with the increase of the blood flow in PAG also. Similarly, the reverse reaction of waiting, anticipation of a painful sensation determines a tendency to inhibition similar to that of an intense stimulation (nocebo effect) [26].

In patients with migraine, interictal, the functional MRI studies revealed an increase in the nociceptive diffuse activity mediated in different ways [27]. Another way of modulating pain is represented by "the nociceptive diffuse control of the pain." The concept, issued by Le Bars since the 8th decade of the last century refers to the wide dynamic range inhibition of neurons from the dorsal horn responsive to a painful stimulation by a nociceptive stimulus applied elsewhere in the body. The inhibition mechanism seems to be central and its loss is involved in the chronic painful syndromes, but also in the becoming chronic and of medication-overuse headache [28, 29]. This system is integrated in the dorsal reticular nucleus which receives nociceptive information from the marrow and communicates with PAG and RVM, amygdala, thalamus, and finally inhibiting the marrow by descending projections. The neurons in dorsal reticular nucleus (DRt) establish connections with the cortex and multiple central nervous system areas involved in modulating the pain–the spino-supraspinatus loop [30].

Perrotta et al. [31] found the existence of a process of central sensitizing of the pain pathways, with the abnormal and facilitating processing of the stimuli in the trigeminal nucleus both in crisis and interictally, suggesting a chronic hyperexcitability possibly conditioned genetically with dysfunctional consequences on the antinociceptive modulating system [32].

It is possible that this demodulation of the nociceptive stimulus processing to be due to a defect of the default mode network, claim supported by the neuroimaging morphofunctional studies which revealed metabolic changes in the brain areas involved in processing the pain. The default mode network consists of a series of relays (part of the medial temporal lobe, part of the medial prefrontal cortex, and the posterior cingulate cortex, along with the adjacent ventral precuneus and the medial, lateral, and inferior parietal cortex) whose anatomical bases are intertwined with the pain processing pathways. The current data suggest that the network is active when the individual is not focused on the outside world and the brain is at wakeful rest and it is possible that it participates in the basic settings of the main brain functions [33].

The hypothalamus, the vegetative brain, establish direct anatomical connections with the trigeminal structures and it is involved in a variety of cerebral functions with vegetative component including regulating the vasomotricity and processing of pain, maintaining the homeostasis. The recent studies have found that there is a disorder of its functional connectivity with the vegetative structures, in the sense of its increasing or decreasing, all being able to disorder the processing of exteroceptive stimuli, especially those painful [34–37].

The hypothalamus is also connected with the sympathetic cerebral structures, such as the parahippocampal gyrus and cerebellar peduncle. The accentuation of connectivity with these centers, found in patients with migraine could prevail in the cortical answer to external nociceptive stimuli. The finding was made by BOLD neuroimaging studies, by increasing the activity in these structures both in sympathetic stimulation and at rest. Similarly, there have been found hyperexcitable connections (enhanced functional connectivity) with parasympathetic structures (temporal pole, superior temporal gyrus, and cerebellar lobules V and VI) ultimately determining a disorder of the processing of internal stimuli in patients with migraine, explaining some features of reaction of the patient to external stimuli [38].

Locus coeruleus, the largest noradrenergic nucleus in the brain is connected by anatomical structures with the hypothalamus, with which it establishes hyperfunctional connections. Involved in modulating the neuronal discharges from thalamus and prefrontal cortex as response to the nociceptive stimuli and in the inhibition of the nociceptive reflexes, it may have an important role in processing the pain in patients with migraine [39]. The caudate nucleus recently involved in processing the pain has also hyperfunctional connectivity with the hypothalamus suggesting an involvement in the chronobiology of migraine [40].

On the other hand, a decrease in the functional connectivity with various cerebral structures (cortical regions in the frontal and occipital regions) was found where hypofunctions were found. No one can say for now that hypothalamus plays in migraine a role similar to vascular face algies, but it certainly interferes with the processing of the pain and it is responsible for a part of the vegetative manifestations in the migraine and their relationship with the human psyche. The disorder could be due to the large amount of information received from the neurons of the spinal trigeminal nucleus, repeated activation during the attacks, and a phenomenon of central sensitizing of the hypothalamic and autonomic connections [41].

In addition to the fast synaptic transmission mediated by classic neurotransmitters, the extra synaptic transmission of chemical signals such as neuropeptides could act a key role for long-term effects following intense noxious stimulation. These extra synaptic peptides, among their intrinsic vascular activity, also increase the excitability of neurons in the dorsal horn and trigger the expression of the immediate-early genes, thus changing the underlying chronicity of the pain.

The transmission of the nerve signal to the trigeminal neurons also involves the presence of some peptides with strong vasodilatory action of the cerebral vessels, the essential link in the pathogenesis of the primary cephalalgias. These peptides (calcitonin gene-related peptide—CGRP, substance P (SP), and neurokinin A—NKA) are often secreted by the same neuron, in different quantities and combinations giving them a remarkable functional diversity. Calcitonin gene-related peptide is the most potent vasodilator transmitter identified in the cerebral circulation, and its action is endothelium independent and associated with an increase in vessel wall cyclic AMP [42–44].

Substance P is a nondecapeptide involved in nociceptive transmission. In many vascular beds, including the cerebral bed, substance P is a potent vasodilator and it also dilates both arteries and veins *in situ* [45]. Substance P can induce protein extravasation in the periphery and a similar response is seen in the dura with protein extravasation and mast cell degranulation [46]. Neurokinin A can relax cerebral vessels both *in vitro* and *in vivo*, although it is only one-tenth as potent as substance P [47]. Both substance P and NKA coexist in perivascular nerve fibers in peripheral and cerebral vessels [48].

It is possible that the antinociceptive system to be activated not only by direct stimulation, but also by disinhibition in PAG. By researching the expression of the protein c-FOS in the activated neurons, patterns different from the neuronal activity in the structures involved in controlling analgesia were found. The existence of these patterns different from the neuronal discharge especially in the spine and finding a background noise have suggested the existence of a tonic activity of the most nociceptive neurons in the posterior horn of the marrow determined by the supraspinal continuous discharges of the endogenous antinociceptive system defining the hypothesis of "prophylactic antinociceptive system" [49].

4. Autonomic system dysfunction in primary headaches

The precise involvement of autonomous nervous system (ANS) in different types of primary headaches is still a subject of debate, as there is still not a clear-cut explanation of the differences found across various studies, both in humans and in animals, concerning the modulation of sympathetic and parasympathetic nervous system. The different results on dysautonomic mechanisms in headache patients can be partially explained by the numerous methods used to quantify the ANS activity, therefore generating specific results for different systems, such as cardiac (e.g., heart rate variability), cardiovascular (e.g., hypotension), pupillary response, and also by the different time-related variations with impact on the vegetative system dynamics [50, 51].

Autonomic dysfunction of different primary headache types have been investigated in several studies, most of them analyzing cardiovascular reflex mechanisms or biochemical changes [52–54]. It is known today that different subtypes of primary headaches share common autonomic mechanisms implying different endogenous molecules and dysfunctional interactions between vegetative pathways and brain-vessel system [55]. Findings indicate as central mechanisms both sympathetic hyperfunction and parasympathetic hypofunction in autonomic manifestations of headache patients [56, 57].

4.1. Sympathetic nervous system and headache

The sympathetic tracts involved in the vascular regulation in headache arise mainly from the ipsilateral superior cervical ganglion, while some nerve fibers that supply the vertebral and basilar arteries originate from the inferior cervical ganglion and the stellate ganglion [58, 59].

The vascular dynamics and regulation of the intracranial pressure are mediated by noradrenaline (NA) and neuropeptide Y (NPY) [60, 61]. Neuropeptide Y is widely distributed throughout sympathetic nerve endings together with NA and it is considered a marker of noradrenergic function. It has been shown that both mediators may be externally influenced, for instance, by sympathectomize, which in turns, stimulates the expression of parasympathetic fibers [62]. NPY participates in the autonomic control of cerebral circulation and can be involved in disorders characterized by neurogenically mediated changes in the cerebral blood flow, such as migraine, cluster headache, and stroke. Decreased NPY concentrations during symptoms-free periods bring further evidence of the dysregulation of the sympathetic function in the course of migraine. The levels of NPY increase during attacks in migraine patients [63]. Microscopic and functional studies have revealed that NPY expression becomes prominent with the increase of sympathetic activity [64]. Furthermore, it has been proven that NA modulates the response of the small pial vessels on the cortical surface and that sympathetic fibers arise from central sources such as locus coeruleus (LC) or the hypothalamus [65–67]. Therefore, via direct influence, destruction of the LC induces a reduction in the number of noradrenergic nerve fibers in intracerebral vessels [59], while on contrary that stimulation of NA neurons in the hypothalamus is associated with an increase in hypothalamic blood flow which is not influenced by superior cervical ganglionectomy or by the β-adrenoceptor antagonist propranolol [68]. These anatomic and physiological features showing central control may represent possible therapeutic targets in primary headaches.

4.2. Parasympathetic nervous system

As it is well known, cerebral blood vessels display perivascular nerves presenting parasympathetic activity (mediated by acetylcholine and acetylcholinesterase activity [69, 70]. The vast majority of parasympathetic nerve fibers to cerebral vessels implied sphenopalatine and otic ganglia [71]. Interesting enough, it has been shown that parasympathetic nerves may interact with sympathetic terminals in the close vicinity of the cerebrovascular smooth muscle effector [71]. Activation of trigeminal nerves and subsequent nociceptive signaling mediates a parasympathetic reflex leading to the release of vasoactive neuropeptides [9, 72, 73]. Vasodilatation of the cranial vessels seems a common property of cranial neurovascular dynamics involving sensory and parasympathetic mechanisms [44, 74].

Along with acetylcholine, there are other neuro messengers that mediate neurogenic vasodilatation, such as vasoactive intestinal peptide (VIP), pituitary adenylate cyclase activating polypeptide (PACAP), and nitric oxide (NO), as demonstrated both by experimental responses of isolated cerebral arteries and by hemodynamic measurements *in vivo* [75–77]. VIP is one of the parasympathetic signaling transmitters contributing to cranial parasympathetic outflow mediated through the sphenopalatine ganglia. It has been shown that VIP coexists with Ach in the perivascular nerve fibers around brain vessels [78]. Although, the VIP-immunoreactive nerve supply is sparse in cerebral arteries or veins, it is considered that VIP concentrations are a marker of parasympathetic activation in migraine [79–81].

4.3. Pathogenic autonomic mechanisms in headache

Large body of data suggests a central role for sensory and parasympathetic mechanisms in the pathophysiology of primary headaches. Studies have provided support for a dysbalance between parasympathetic and sympathetic nervous system, which trigger the pathogenic mechanisms and contribute to the clinical presentation in primary headaches. The activation of the parasympathetic cranial outflow during migraine and cluster headache (CH) attacks seems to be due to the activation of the trigeminovascular system, which was described previously. This implies the release of specific neuromediators, such as the neuropeptide calcitonin gene-related peptide (CGRP) [82].

Some studies used transcranial Doppler sonography to assess vascular oscillations corresponding to myogenic cerebrovascular regulation in migraine and tension-headache patients [55, 83]. Most of the data focus on migraine, a chronic neurovascular disorder, which is classically considered the result of the sympathetic system unbalance, generally meaning increased sympathetic activity, although some studies showed decreased sympathetic activity [53, 57]. Both in the prodromal phase and in the headache phase of a migrainous episode, there are vegetative symptoms, such as hunger, sleepiness, and orthostatic hypotension initially, and later, in the headache phase, vomiting and nausea, pointing out a close relationship between the ANS and this type of headache [2]. The autonomic manifestations imply decreased plasma noradrenaline levels and increased adrenergic receptor sensitivity [53]. There are still contradictory data on the exact involvement of sympathetic system in migraine. Some studies investigated cardiac and cardiovascular reactions during vagal and sympathetic activation [84]. An increased basal sympathetic tone is also suggested by a frequent association of hypertension with migraine [85]. However, the association of migraine with blood pressure variations is still unclear, as there are studies showing an increased diastolic blood pressure in migraine and also an association of migraine with lower blood pressure [85]. Sympathetic hypofunction has been reported for migraine in studies of pupil diameter [82, 86], cardiovascular reflex responses, and heart rate recovery [87]. The heart rate variability in migraine patients across a longer time period was different compared to healthy controls during normal daily activity, which pointed out parasympathetic hypofunction in migraine patients [88].

Sympathetic skin responses [89] and salivary amylase levels as marker of sympathoadrenal medullary activity [90] seem decreased during migraine attacks, suggesting the dynamic involvement of the sympathetic system in this pathology.

Gass and Glaros [91] examined different vegetative biomarkers such as the heart rate variability, skin temperature, skin conductance, and respiration in patients with migraine and compared to healthy controls, and found in migraine patients a decreased variability of the consecutive R-to-R intervals, therefore pleading for a sympathetic hyperfunction and decreased parasympathetic tone in migraine patients [91]. Yerdelen et al. [87] examined heart rate recovery after physical exercise as an index for vagal parasympathetic activity in migraine and tension-type headache patients (TTH) and controls and showed that even though parasympathetic function has not been affected in migraine and TTH patients, sympathetic tone in migraine patients is elevated compared to patients with episodic tension-type headache [87].

In an interesting study, Tomé-Pires and Miró [92] measured skin conductance responses (SCRs) in migraine versus control subjects while presenting pain descriptors, emotional negative words, and neutral words [92]. The authors showed no differences in the skin conductance responses in the two groups, but migraineurs recalled more emotional words than controls, thus suggesting possible new avenues to modulate migraine pain perception and autonomic responses.

4.4. Cluster headache

This type of headache implies the ophthalmic division of the trigeminal nerve responsible for the pain manifestations. In addition, there are signs of parasympathetic over activity acting on the facial and cranial vasculature, such as lacrimation, nasal congestion, and injection of the eyes [2]. Cranial parasympathetic systems may be involved in mediating these dysfunctions, with the release of the VIP stimulating vasomotor facial symptoms [93]. Furthermore, it has been shown that noxious chemical stimulation of rat facial mucosa increases intracranial blood flow through a trigemino-parasympathetic reflex, which may explain the involvement of autonomic pathway [94]. Animal models used superior salivatory nucleus as a model to measure cranial autonomic symptoms and changes in blood flow in the lacrimal gland/duct as a measure of cranial autonomic activation [95]. The superior salivatory nucleus projects to the cranial vessels through the sphenopalatine ganglion, via the greater pietrosal nerve of the facial nerve. Electrophysiological methods measured neural activity in response to superior salivatory nucleus stimulation. There were two populations of neurons with differential latencies in action. The longer latency neuronal response was mediated by activation of the parasympathetic outflow and that the action of oxygen—as the therapeutic approach, is likely via this pathway. The shorter latency response seemed most likely via antidromic activation of the trigeminal autonomic reflex [96]. Moreover, it has been shown also that posterior hypothalamus may play a central role in the CH, thus explaining the circadian and circannual periodicity of the symptoms [97].

4.5. Tension-type headache (TTH)

Although very frequent, the relationship between the tension-type headache and ANS activity is less documented [87]. It seems that chronic TTH along with migraine may be associated with increased sympathetic tonus, expressed by elevated resting heart rate, compared to episodic TTH [93]. TTH patients may also have a delayed adaptation in heart-rate to stress and a reduced pain control system inhibition [97].

Even though the dynamics of ANS intervention in primary headaches is not yet fully understood, the emergence of translational research models and also the development of new techniques to measure the vegetative biomarkers in headaches provide a robust basis for new and more efficient therapeutic strategies.

5. Heart rate variability as a measure of autonomic nervous system in migraine

The autonomic nervous system (ANS) has important functions in maintaining homeostasis by adjustment of the body to internal and environmental demands. Beside key functions controlled by the ANS such as respiration, blood pressure, heart rate, hormonal regulation, etc., ANS is also involved in regulating emotional behavior and cognitive functions.

The sympathetic nervous system (SNS) controls of the heart coming from the upper thoracic region of the spinal cord. Preganglionic fibers synapse with postganglionic sympathetic fibers and release acetylcholine, which binds to nicotinic receptors on the postganglionic fibers. Through sympathetic adrenergic efferent fibers extend to the sinoatrial and atrioventricular nodes in the heart where they release norepinephrine at synapses with beta-adrenergic receptors [98]. Stimulation of the SNS increases heart rate (positive chronotropy), ventricular contraction (positive inotropy), conduction velocity (positive dromotropy), and rate of relaxation (positive lusitropy). The parasympathetic nervous system (PNS) control of the heart coming from vagal nuclei within the medulla oblongata in the brainstem, and efferent nervous outflow occurs via the 10th cranial nerve (vagus nerve). The long preganglionic efferent nerve fibers extent to the heart and synapse with a ganglia located near the sinoatrial and atrioventricular nodes. Acetylcholine is released, binds to nicotinic receptors, and activates short postganglionic efferent nerve fibers. These postganglionic fibers synapses with muscarinic receptors in the sinoatrial and atrioventricular nodes, and is activated by acetylcholine. For heart PNS decreases heart rate (negative chronotropy), force of atrial contraction (negative inotropy), rate of relaxation (negative lusitropy), and negative dromotropy [98].

The actions of the SNS and PNS are often opposing in their effects and normally the SNS and PNS activities are in dynamic balance thus indicating a healthy and flexible physiological system [99]. The autonomic imbalance described by increased SNS activity and suppressed PNS activity is associated with an increased risk of diseases [99]. The central control of cardiovascular system involved several areas throughout spinal, bulbopontine, pontomesencephalic, and forebrain. The medullary centers work through reflex cardiovascular mechanisms such as baroreflex, chemoreflex, and cardiopulmonary reflex [100]. The afferent fibers of the cardiovascular reflexes are terminated in the nucleus tractus solitarii [100]. The reticular formation of the ventrolateral medulla (VLM) is the primary central site that regulates sympathetic outflow, thus contributing to the regulation of BP and heart rate (HR). In the rostral VLM part are excitatory neurons which synapse in the intermediolateral gray column of the spinal cord, and in the caudal VLM are inhibitory neurons that sent projections to the rostral VLM. The preganglionic parasympathetic neurons located in the nucleus ambiguous and the dorsal motor nucleus of vagus are involved in the parasympathetic regulation of the cardiac reflexes [101]. Also parabrachial nucleus, Kolliker-Fuse nucleus, the cluster of A5 cells are the brainstem centers involved in the control of the cardiovascular system.

The upper brainstem level includes the periaqueductal gray matter (PAG), which integrates the autonomic control with pain modulation and behavioral responses to stress [102]. The forebrain level includes the paraventricular and related nuclei of the hypothalamus, thalamus, amygdala, and anterior cingulate cortex, the insular and medial prefrontal cortex that integrates autonomic and endocrine responses [102]. The anterior limbic circuit (insula, the anterior cingulate cortex, and amygdala) assures integration of specific sensations with emotional and goal-related autonomic responses [102]. Electrical stimulation of the prefrontal and cingulate cortex, left insula, lateral nucleus of hypothalamus decreased heart rate and blood pressure, whereas electrical stimulation of right insula, ventromedial nucleus of hypothalamus increased heart rate and blood pressure [103]. Stimulation of the basolateral nucleus of amygdala increases blood pressure and decreases heart rate; stimulation of the rostral nucleus of amygdala results in depressor effects and variable changes in heart rate [103].

The normal sympathovagal regulation induces an increase in heart rate during inspiration and decrease during expiration, and this physiological phenomenon is known as respiratory arrhythmia. The intrinsic heart rate is 105 beats/minute while resting heart rate is only 60–80 beats/minute, indicating that the heart is under "vagal dominance" [104].

The electrical signal produced by the heart can be measured with an electrocardiogram. Electrocardiogram registers depolarization of the atria (P-wave), depolarization of the ventricles (the QRS complex), and repolarization of the ventricles (T-wave). Using these points we can measure heart period or inter beat interval which measure the time between two consecutive heart beats in milliseconds [105]. Heart rate (HR) measures the numbers of consecutive heart beats in 1 min (beats per min). The analysis of consecutive sinus rhythm R-R intervals is known as heart rate variability (HRV), a noninvasive electrocardiographic marker reflecting the activity of the ANS on sinus node function.

HRV parameters can be calculated in time domain (statistical and geometrical), frequency domain (power spectral density), and nonlinear measures. In time domain methods HRV parameters are standard deviation between normal intervals during recording—SDNN (ms), standard deviation of the average values of NN intervals calculated from all 5-min segments of the entire recording—SDANN (ms), square root of the mean of the sum of the squares of differences between adjacent NN intervals—RMSSD (ms), percentage of differences between adjacent NN intervals differing more than 50 ms—pNN50% [105]. A lot of studies indicate that SDNN, RMSSD, and pNN50%, time domain indicators of the HRV, represent the activity of the vagal nerve.

Using simultaneously the Fast Fourier transform method and parametric– autoregressive method (AR), HRV can be analyzed in frequency domain (power spectral analyses of HRV) in which can be measured low-frequency component ($LF < 0.15$ Hz) taken as an indicator of both vagal and sympathetic functions, high-frequency component ($HF \geq 0.15$ Hz) as an indicator of parasympathetic function, very low-frequency component (VLF—the frequency band in the range 0.003–0.04 Hz), ultra-low-frequency (ULF—the frequency band below 0.003 Hz), and the total power (TP) [105, 106]. VLF is related to the thermoregulatory sympathetic vascular activity and to oscillations in the renin-angiotensin system [107]. The ratio of LF/HF is considered as an index of cardiac sympathetic/parasympathetic tone balance.

Abnormalities in the SNS or PNS have been found in migraine patients during the headache-free phase [108, 109]. Some researchers revealed sympathetic hypofunction and parasympathetic hyper-function in migraine patients during the same period [83, 110]. Other study found that older patients with migraine may have sympathetic hyper-function and a parasympathetic hypofunction during headache-free intervals [111]. Martin et al. [112] found a reduction of HR during deep breathing, and after 2 min of tilting. Appel et al. [113] revealed increase of the low-frequency band of HRV analysis in migraineurs, suggesting an increase in sympathetic activity.

We tried to analyze the ANS involvement in migraine using the HRV on long-term 24-h ECG. We investigated 27 subjects with migraine (10 with migraine with aura and 17 without aura) during headache-free periods and 10 age-matched healthy control subjects. We found a significant decrease in SDNN, RMSSD, and HF indicating parasympathetic dysfunction in migraine groups during night headache-free periods, and the most affected were migraine with aura patients (**Figures 1** and **2**). LF and LF/HF ratio were increased during the night in migraine with aura patients (**Figures 3** and **4**). In both groups of migraine patients, we discovered an autonomic nervous system dysfunction. The most marked ANS impairment being present in the group of migraine with aura sufferers where we found sympathetic hyperfunction associated with parasympathetic hypofunction especially at night with loss of circadian rhythms [114].

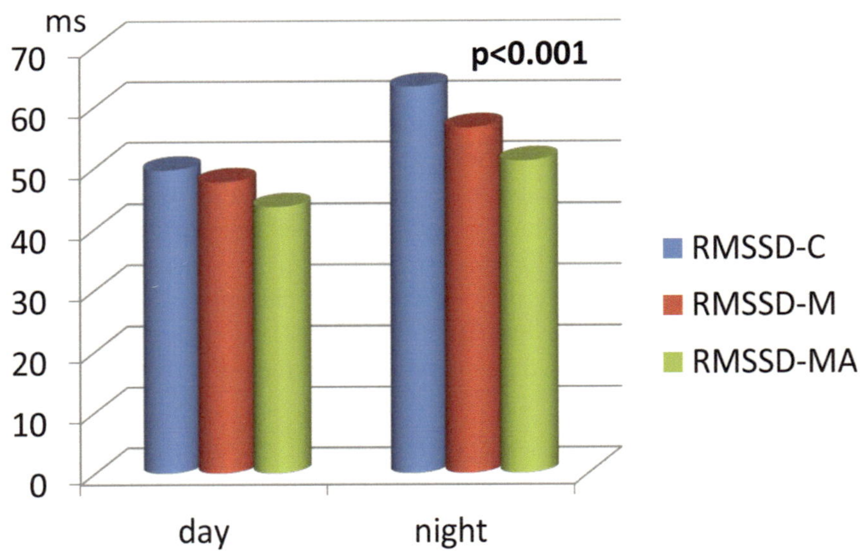

Figure 1. Square root of the mean of the sum of the squares of differences between adjacent NN intervals—RMSSD (ms) in study groups (C, control group; M, migraine without aura group, MA, migraine with aura group).

http://dx.doi.org/10.5772/65737

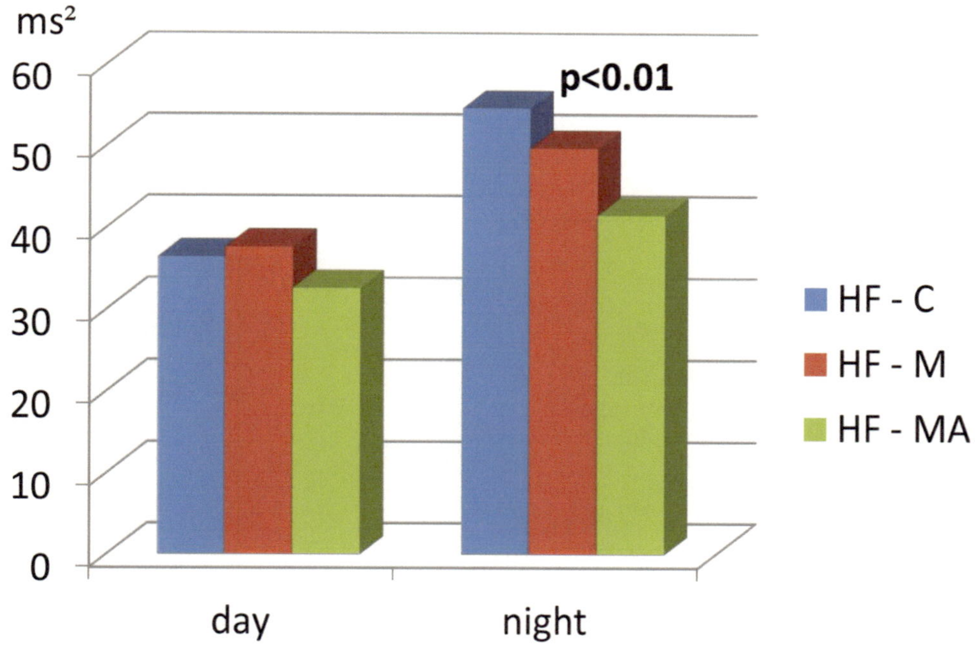

Figure 2. High-frequency component of power spectral analyses of HRV in study groups.

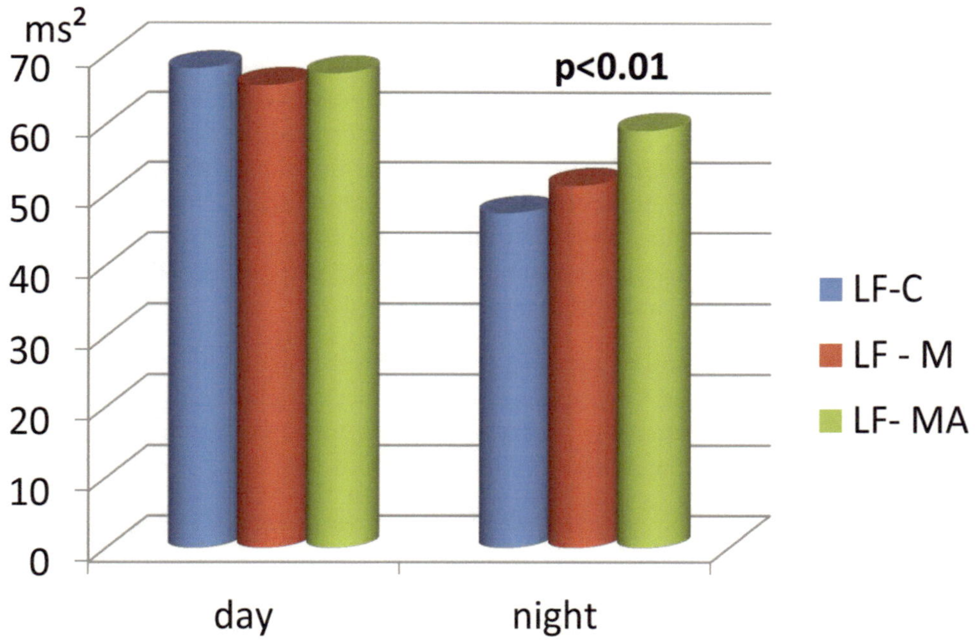

Figure 3. Low-frequency component of power spectral analyses of HRV in study groups.

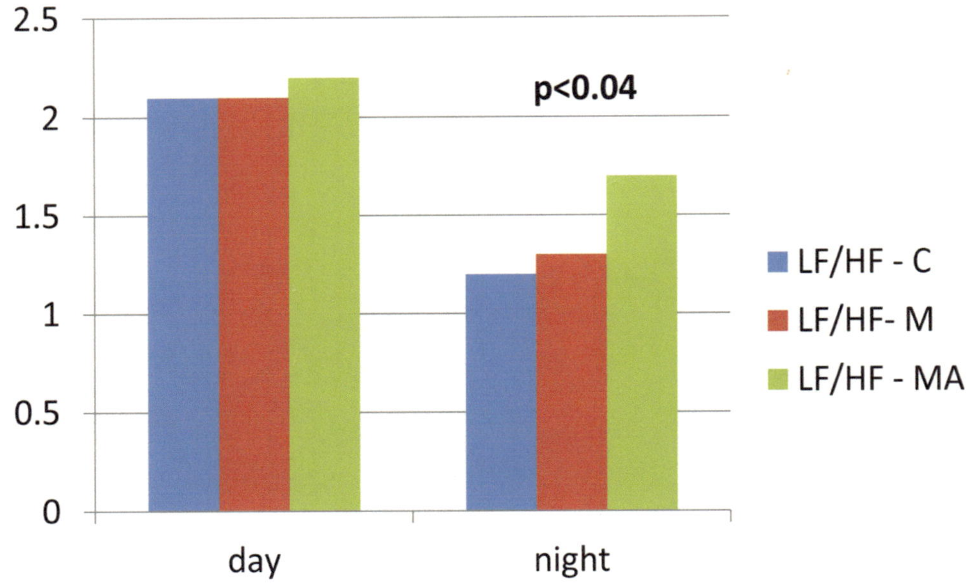

Figure 4. LF/HF ratio in study groups.

HRV is associated with highly functional prefrontal cortex inhibitory activity over subcortical structures that make the body to well adapt to the environment. Low HRV is associated with reduced prefrontal inhibitory control over subcortical structures and failure to recognize safety signals [104]. Failure of inhibition leads to continue to process fear information and is linked with anxiety and depression [115]. Chronic psychological stress and depressed mood have been shown to be associated with SNS dominance and vagal withdrawal, highlighted by decreased HRV [115, 116]. In our study, we found an increased frequency of anxiety and depressive symptoms in migraine patients, especially in migraine with aura group [114]. Individuals with high level of stress, anxiety, and depression display an imbalance between PNS and SNS activities. Prolonged stress may influence health via several different pathways, i.e., alterations in autonomic nervous system (increased SNS and decrease PNS), neuroendocrine activity, immune, behavioral, and cognitive functions.

Many other factors such as alcohol, nicotine, physical exercise, age, gender, diabetes, hypertension, cardiovascular disease, sleep apnea, chronic respiratory disease, or medications (sex steroid hormones, antidepressants, μ- blockers, etc.) may influence the autonomic nervous system [117–121]. Moreover, the ANS exhibits a circadian variation [122].

The ANS involvement during the premonitory phase of a migraine attack is suggested by many symptoms and signs with potential involvement of the hypothalamus (depression, irritability, fatigue, food cravings, and increase yawning), brainstem (neck stiffness), and cortex (abnormal sensitivity to light, sound, and smell) [123]. Nausea, vomiting, dizziness, cutaneous vasoconstriction or vasodilation, conjunctival injection, lacrimation, nasal congestion, rhinorrhea, eyelid edema, piloerection, and diaphoresis can occur during pain phase [108, 109]. Also accompanying psychological and cognitive symptoms can appear—inability to organize thoughts and plans, physical exhaustion, confusion, agitation, aggressiveness, depression, and anxiety.

Migraine can be initiated by diverse triggers including bright lights, sounds, hunger, and mental exertion; poor sleep quality, menses, excess consumption of alcohol, chocolate, and fermented cheese. Sleep usually calms the pain.

In our study when we asked patients about sleep quality and dreaming, they complained about bad sleep quality. The majority experience negative sensations such as anxiety, fear, or terror and contents such as perception of fall and unsuccessful efforts to do various things [114]. These observations suggest that there is some malfunction in the prefrontal cortex, limbic system, amygdala, and hypothalamus, elements involved in dream and migraine pathophysiology [124]. Activation of the limbic system, amygdala, and anterior cingulate cortex observed in rapid eye movement sleep are involved in cardiovascular regulation and could reflect responses to intense emotions such as fear and anxiety found in migraine patients during night [125].

When physiological stressors, such as migraine attacks, are frequent and persistent allostatic responses can become maladaptive, resulting in changes of the body system. Migraine patients were found to have elevated plasma levels of cortisol in headache-free periods [126] and during pain period [127]. Increased chronic levels of cortisol can induce atrophy in the PFC, decrease dopamine in the brain pleasure circuits, deplete the norepinephrine from the LC, and reduce frontal lobe serotonin receptors levels, thus contributing to flatness of emotion, concentration weakening, mood dysfunctions, and bad quality of sleep [128]. Neurogenesis and apoptosis in hippocampus are suppressed [129] and also dysregulation of the autonomic nervous system and hypothalamic-pituitary-adrenal axis with alterations in hormone regulation are revealed during chronic stress. Chronic migraineurs show decreased amygdala volume [130] that can be related to the high levels of anxiety or fear in these patients [131]. In chronic migraine, beside cortisol, other dysfunction in hormone secretion has been reported for prolactin, and melatonin [132]. Sleep deprivation and circadian disruption can have negative consequences for body functions including increased appetite, increased levels of proinflammatory cytokines, decreased parasympathetic and increased sympathetic tone, increased blood pressure, and elevated insulin and blood glucose [133]. Hormonal dysfunctions in estrogen and progesterone regulation are frequent in migraine patients, and migraine improves after menopause or with hormonal therapies [134].

The cumulative effects of migraine over the body, as well as its treatment represents allostatic load [135]. Early interruption of a feed-forward vicious cycle with different techniques (medication and stress reduction) is important to diminish allostatic load [135].

6. New directions in the treatment of primary headaches

It is classically accepted that migraine may respond to few different pharmacological agents such as pain-relieving medications (like triptans) in acute phase and preventive medication like antiepileptics (like topiramate), CH responds to oxygen and parenteral triptans, while verapamil has the most success for prevention. Paroxysmal hemicrania responds to indomethacin. SUNCT/SUNA responds to lamotrigine and topiramate. Hemicrania continua respond to indomethacin [136].

6.1. Neurostimulation

A promising and rather new venue in headache treatment seems to be represented by neuromodulation of pain central system and autonomic pathways. These noninvasive methods may provide relief in patients with chronic and pharmacoresistant forms of headache. Therefore, it was reported that transcutaneous stimulation of the parasympathetic nerve system via the vagus nerve can abort migraine attacks [137]. Vagal nerve stimulation represents a well-established nonpharmacological strategy in epileptic patients with intractable seizures and also in depressed patients. Some cohorts of epileptic patients with implanted VNS have shown improvement in their migraine symptoms, but the eventual causality with seizure frequency reduction still needs to be debated also [138]. Similarly, patients known with migraine and treated with VNS for depression experienced an improvement in the migraine attacks [139]. Yet, further studies need to clarify the exact correlation between VNS effects and migraine mechanisms.

Recently, it has been shown that patients with CH seem also to benefit from noninvasive VNS, with improvement of their initial condition of approximately 50% [140]. On the other hand, occipital nerve stimulation (ONS) has proved favorable clinical results in the treatment of refractory chronic CH in well-documented cases, but there are still limited studies in this direction. The hypothalamic activation during cluster attacks led to the introduction of deep brain stimulation (DBS) technique for refractory CH, with rather positive effects. Still, there is need of further confirmation of this method in CH, in terms of targeted anatomo-functional centers and patients selection in order to have a good risk/benefit outcome [141, 142].

6.2. Modulation of signaling molecules

Migraine is considered as a syndrome of chronically low central serotonin system with consequent 5-HT receptor hypersensitivity, with migraine attacks triggered by a sudden increase in 5-HT release [143]. Therefore, medication targeting specific serotoninergic pathways showed its efficiency in migraine acute treatment. Triptans are selective serotonin agonists, specifically acting at 5-hydroxytryptamine 1B/1D/1F (5-HT1B/1D/1F) receptors on intracranial blood vessels and sensory nerve endings. The first combination product of a triptan and a nonsteroid anti-inflammatory drug (naproxen) was approved by the U.S. Food and Drug Administration in April 2008. It has been proven that migraineurs who experienced poor response to a short-acting triptan, the combination of sumatriptan/naproxen sodium reported more effective results in pain reduction and migraine-associated symptoms of photophobia and phonophobia [144].

New prevention strategy via biochemical signaling in migraine prevention is based on monoclonal calcitonin gene-related peptide (CGRP) antibodies to CGRP are effective in

http://dx.doi.org/10.5772/65737

migraine prophylaxis [145]. As shown previously, robust data showed that neuropeptides present in the perivascular space of cranial vessels are important mediators of nociceptive input during migraine attacks. Pituitary adenylate cyclase-activating polypeptide (PACAP) is present in sensory trigeminal neurons and may modulate nociception at different levels of the nervous system. It has been proposed that the PAC(1) receptor represents a possible signaling pathway implicated in migraine and may be a future pharmacological target in migraine treatment [146].

The precise implication of the hypothalamus in premonitory phases of migraine and also during migraine attacks is discussed. Therefore, novel targets may include hypothalamic peptides such as orexine, which interferes with trigeminal nociceptive activity and cortical spreading depression–the well-known neural phenomena in the prodromal phase of migraine [147]. Interestingly, Botulinum toxin A was associated with a small or modest benefit for chronic daily headaches and chronic migraines, reducing headache episodes per month [148].

6.3. Genetic therapies

Genetic studies have highlighted a potential role in the etiopathogenesis of primary headaches for several genes related to vascular, neuronal, and neuroendocrine mechanisms. Therefore, recent data showed the implication of new genes, like methylenetetrahydrofolate reductase (MTHFR), potassium channel, subfamily K member 18 (KCNK18), transient related potential vanilloid type 1 (TRPV1), transient related potential vanilloid type 3 (TRPV3), hypocretin (orexin) receptor 1 (HCRTR1), and hypocretin (orexin) receptor 2 (HCRTR2), both in migraine and cluster headache. Of course, further preclinical and clinical data need to confirm the precise place and indication of genetic intervention when addressing primary headaches, thus promoting the multifactorial determination of this pathology [149].

6.4. Multidisciplinary nonpharmacological interventions

Behavioral and psychological coaching in chronic headache patients in a multidisciplinary setting may foster treatment adherence and improve the quality of life in these patients. It is considered that behavioral therapy combined with pharmacological intervention (for example, beta blocker alone) renders more effective treatment [150].

The above-mentioned directions of treatment in primary headache highlight the complexity of the pathogenic mechanisms of this pathology and the need for further studies to address therapeutic strategies adapted to individual condition.

7. Conclusions

Headache disorders represent both a treatment challenge and a serious public health concern, with major impact on the individual and society. Although the painful symptomatology is the main encounter for the decreased quality of life and discomfort, the vegetative manifestations which frequently accompany the cephalalgic syndromes, cause an important amount of distress. Despite the advancement of the understanding of the molecular basis of headache disorders and neurovascular complex interactions, both at central and peripheral levels, especially concerning migraine, there is still lack of an integrated view of the neurovegetative modulation in different types of primary cephalalgic syndromes, translating from animal pathophysiologic "models" to clinical data. As shown in this chapter, the neurochemical mechanisms which subtend dysautonomic manifestations in different types of headache share common pathways, yet there is need to specifically address the various vegetative biomarkers in each type of headache, in order to provide more efficient and individualized therapeutic strategies, combining multimodal pharmacological and nonpharmacological approaches.

Without pretending exhaustively, this chapter highlights the need for a better and a more accurate characterization and classification of primary headaches, taking into consideration the whole spectrum of clinical manifestations, including the dysautonomic activity. Despite locally derived, population-based data describing the burden of primary headache disorders, there is still need of a global perspective on disease impact, through both preclinical and clinical data, in both developed and developing countries, in order to maximize efforts for a better understanding and management of the disease.

Acknowledgements

This work was supported by "Grigore T. Popa" University of Medicine and Pharmacy Iasi. Authors contributed equally to this work.

conflict of interest

The authors confirm that this chapter contents have no conflict of interest.

Author details

Cuciureanu Dan Iulian[1], Constantinescu Irina[1], Constantinescu Victor[1], Corciova Calin[2] and Matei Daniela[2*]

*Address all correspondence to: dvm2202@yahoo.com

1 Department of Neurology, Faculty of Medicine, "Grigore T. Popa" University of Medicine and Pharmacy, Iasi, Romania

2 Department of Biomedical Sciences, Faculty of Medical Bioengineering, "Grigore T. Popa" University of Medicine and Pharmacy, Iasi, Romania

References

[1] World Health Organization, http://www.who.int/mediacentre/factsheets

[2] Headache Classification Committee of the International Headache Society. The International Classification of Headache Disorders, 3rd edition (beta version). Cephalalgia. 2013; 33(9):629–808. doi: 10.1177/0333102413485658

[3] Keller JT, Marfurt CF. Peptidergic and serotoninergic innervation of the rat dura mater. J Comp Neurol. 1991; 309(4):515–534. doi:10.1002/cne.903090408

[4] Levy D, Strassman AM. Mechanical response properties of A and C primary afferent neurons innervating the rat intracranial dura. J Neurophysiol. 2002; 88(6):3021–3031. doi: 10.1152/jn.00029.2002

[5] Steiger HJ, Meakin CJ. The meningeal representation in the trigeminal ganglion–an experimental study in the cat. Headache. 1984; 24:305–309.

[6] Messlinger K. Functional morphology of nociceptive and other fine sensory endings (free nerve endings) in different tissues. In: The polymodal Receptor: A Gateway to Pathological Pain, Elsevier, Amsterdam, 1996; pp. 273–298.

[7] Suzuki N, Hardebo JE. The pathway of parasympathetic nerve fibers to cerebral vessels from the otic gangl ion in the rat. J Auton Nerv Syst. 1991; 36:39–46.

[8] Edvinsson L, Uddman R. Adrenergic, cholinergic and peptidergic nerve fibres in dura mater–involvement in headache? Cephalalgia Int J Headache. 1981; 1:175–179.

[9] Hardebo JE, Arbab M, Suzuki N, Svendgaard NA. Pathways of parasympathetic and sensory cerebrovascular nerves in monkeys. Stroke. 1991; 22(3):331–42.

[10] Moskowitz MA, Buzzi MG. Neuroeffector functions of sensory fibres: implications for headache mechanisms and drug actions. J Neurol. 1991; 238(Suppl 1):S18–S22.

[11] Schwedt TJ, Schlaggar BL, Mar S, Nolan T, Coalson RS, Nardos B, Benzinger T, Larson-Prior LJ. Atypical resting-state functional connectivity of affective pain regions in chronic migraine. Headache. 2013; 53(5):737–751. doi: 10.1111/head.12081

[12] DaSilva AF, Granziera C, Snyder J, Hadjikhani N. Thickening in the somatosensory cortex of patients with migraine. Neurology. 2007; 69(21):1990–1995. doi: 10.1212/01.wnl.0000291618.32247.2d

[13] Upadhyay J, Knudsen J, Anderson J, Becerra L, Borsook D. Noninvasive mapping of human trigeminal brainstem pathways. Magn Reson Med. 2008; 60:1037–1046. doi: 10.1002/mrm.21682

[14] Stankewitz A, Voit HL, Bingel U, Peschke C, May A. A new trigemino-nociceptive stimulation model for event-related Fmri. Cephalalgia. 2010; 30(4):475–485. doi: 10.1111/j.1468-2982.2009.01968.x

[15] Krause P, Förderreuther S, Straube A. Motor cortical representation in patients with complex regional pain syndrome: a TMS study. Schmerz. 2006; 20(3):181–184, 186–188. doi: 10.1007/s00482-005-0417-8

[16] Ter Laan M, van Dijk JM, Elting JW, Staal MJ, Absalom AR. Sympathetic regulation of cerebral blood flow in humans: a review. Br J Anaesth. 2013; 111(3):361–367. doi: 10.1093/bja/aet122.

[17] Tracey I, Johns E. The pain matrix: reloaded or reborn as we image tonic pain using arterial spin labelling. Pain. 2010; 148(3):359–360. doi: 10.1016/j.pain.2009.11.009

[18] Neugebauer V, Galhardo V, Maione S, Mackey SC. Forebrain pain mechanisms. Brain Res Rev. 2009; 60(1):226–242. doi: 10.1016/j.brainresrev.2008.12.014.

[19] Fields HL, Anderson SD, Clanton CH, Basbaum AI. Nucleus raphe magnus: a common mediator of opiate-and stimulus-produced analgesia. Trans Am Neurol Assoc. 1976; 101:208–210.

[20] Meng ID, Johansen JP, Harasawa I, Fields HL. Kappa opioids inhibit physiologically identified medullary pain modulating neurons and reduce morphine antinociception. J Neurophysiol. 2005; 93(3):1138–1144. doi: 10.1152/jn.00320.2004

[21] Heinricher MM, Barbaro NM, Fields HL. Putative nociceptive modulating neurons in the rostral ventromedial medulla of the rat: firing of on-and off-cells is related to nociceptive responsiveness. Somatosens Mot Res. 1989; 6(4):427–439. 48–50

[22] Mainero C, Zhang WT, Kumar A, Rosen BR, Sorensen AG. Mapping the spinal and supraspinal pathways of dynamic mechanical allodynia in the human trigeminal system using cardiac-gated fMRI. Neuroimage. 2007; 35:1201–1210. doi: 10.1016/j.neuroimage.2007.01.024

[23] Gassner M, Ruscheweyh R, Sandkuhler J. Direct excitation of spinal GABAergic interneurons by noradrenaline. Pain. 2009; 145(1–2):204–210. doi: 10.1016/j.pain.2009.06.021

[24] McCorry LK editor. Essentials of Human Physiology for Pharmacy, 2nd ed. CRC Press, Pharmacy Education series. 2008; p.99–100. ISBN-13: 978-1420043907 ISBN-10: 1420043900

[25] Sandkühler J. The organization and function of endogenous antinociceptive systems. Prog Neurobiol. 1996; 50(1):49–81.

[26] Benedetti F, Lanotte M, Lopiano L, Colloca L. When words are painful: unraveling the mechanisms of the nocebo effect. NeuroScience. 2007; 147(2):260–271. doi: 10.1016/j.neuroscience.2007.02.020

[27] Russo A, Tessitore A, Esposito F, Marcuccio L, Giordano A, Conforti R, Truini A, Paccone A, d'Onofrio F, Tedeschi G. Pain processing in patients with migraine: an event-

related fMRI study during trigeminal nociceptive stimulation. J Neurol. 2012; 259(9): 1903–1912.

[28] Villanueva L. Diffuse noxious inhibitory control (DNIC) as a tool for exploring dysfunction of endogenous pain modulatory systems. Pain. 2009; 143(3):161–162. doi: 10.1016/j.pain.2009.03.003

[29] Okada-Ogawa A, Porreca F, Meng ID. Sustained morphine-induced sensitization and loss of diffuse noxious inhibitory controls in dura-sensitive medullary dorsal horn neurons. J Neurosci. 2009; 29(50):15828–15835. doi: 10.1523/JNEUROSCI.3623-09.2009

[30] Le Bars D. The whole body receptive field of dorsal horn multireceptive neurones. Brain Res Brain Res Rev. 2002; 40(1–3):29–44.

[31] Perrotta A, Serrao M, Ambrosini A, Bolla M, Coppola G, Sandrini G, Pierelli F. Facilitated temporal processing of pain and defective supraspinal control of pain in cluster headache. Pain. 2013; 154(8):1325–1332. doi: 10.1016/j.pain.2013.04.012

[32] Ayzenberg I, Obermann M, Nyhuis P, Gastpar M, Limmroth V, Diener HC, Kaube H, Katsarava Z. Central sensitization of the trigeminal and somatic nociceptive systems in medication overuse headache mainly involves cerebral supraspinal structures. Cephalalgia. 2006; 26(9):1106–1114. doi: 10.1111/j.1468-2982.2006.01183.x

[33] Perrotta A. Pain processing in primary headaches, from spinal sensitisation to cortical modulation. J Headache Pain. 2015; 16(Suppl 1):A12. doi: 10.1186/1129-2377-16-S1-A12

[34] Lambru G, Matharu MS. Trigeminal autonomic cephalalgias: A review of recent diagnostic, therapeutic and pathophysiological developments, Ann Indian Acad Neurol. 2012; 15(Suppl 1):S51–S61. doi: 10.4103/0972-2327.100007

[35] Malick A, Burstein R. Cells of origin of the trigeminohypothalamic tract in the rat. J Comp Neurol. 1998; 400(1):125–144.

[36] Goadsby PJ. Trigeminal autonomic cephalalgias: fancy term or constructive change to the IHS classification? J Neurol Neurosurg Psychiatry. 2005; 76:301–305.

[37] Bartsch T, Levy MJ, Knight YE, Goadsby PJ. Differential modulation of nociceptive dural input to [hypocretin] Orexin A and B receptor activation in the posterior hypothalamic area. Pain. 2004; 109:367–378. doi: 10.1016/j.pain.2004.02.005

[38] Moulton EA, Becerra L, Johnson A, Burstein R, Borsook D. Altered hypothalamic functional connectivity with autonomic circuits and the locus coeruleus in migraine. PLoS One. 2014; 9(4):e95508. doi:10.1371/journal.pone.0095508

[39] Condes-Lara M. Different direct pathways of locus coeruleus to medial prefrontal cortex and centrolateral thalamic nucleus: electrical stimulation effects on the evoked responses to nociceptive peripheral stimulation. Eur J Pain. 1998; 2:15–23. doi: 10.1016/S1090-3801(98)90042-8

[40] Borsook D, Upadhyay J, Chudler EH, Becerra L. A key role of the basal ganglia in pain and analgesia–insights gained through human functional imaging. Mol Pain. 2010; 6:27. doi: 10.1186/1744-8069-6-27

[41] Burstein R, Jakubowski M. Unitary hypothesis for multiple triggers of the pain and strain of migraine. J Comp Neurol. 2005; 493:9–14. doi: 10.1002/cne.20688

[42] Edvinsson L, Fredholm BB, Hamel E, Jansen I, Verrecchia C. Perivascular peptides relax cerebral arteries concomitant with stimulation of cyclic adenosine monophosphate accumulation of release of an endothelium-derived relaxing factor in the cat. Neurosci Lett. 1985; 58:213–217. doi: 10.1016/0304-3940(85)90166-1

[43] Amara SG, Jonas V, Rosenfeld MG, Ong ES, Evans RM. Alternative RNA processing in calcitonin gene expression generates mRNAs encoding different polypeptide products. Nature. 1982; 298:240–244. doi: 10.1038/298240a0

[44] May A, Goadsby PJ. The trigeminovascular system in humans: pathophysiologic implications for primary headache syndromes of the neural influences on the cerebral circulation. J Cereb Blood Flow Metab. 1999; 19(2):115–27.

[45] Edvinsson L, McCulloch J, Uddman R. Substance P: immunohistochemical localization and effect upon cat pial arteries in vitro and in situ. J Physiol. 1981; 318:251–258.

[46] Moskowitz MA, Cutrer FM. Sumatriptan: a receptor-targeted treatment for migraine. Ann Rev Med. 1993; 44:145–154. doi: 10.1146/annurev.me.44.020193.001045

[47] Jansen I, Alafaci C, McCulloch J, Uddman R, Edvinsson L. Tachykinins (substance P, neurokinin A, neuropeptide K, and neurokinin B) in the cerebral circulation: vasomotor responses in vitro and in situ. J Cereb Blood Flow Metab. 1991; 11:567–575. doi: 10.1038/jcbfm.1991.105

[48] Sundler F, Brodin E, Ekblad E, Hakanson R, Uddman R. Sensory nerve fibers: distribution of substance P, neurokinin A and calcitonin gene-related peptide. In: Tachykinin Antagonists (Hakanson R, Sundler F, eds.), Elsevier, Amsterdam, 1985; pp. 3–14.

[49] Sandkühler J. Endogenous analgesic mechanism: new concepts from functional neuroanatomy, neurophysiology, neurobiology and chaos research. Schmerz. 1993; 7(4):250–261. doi: 10.1007/BF02529861

[50] Buzzi MG, Bonamini M, Cerbo R. The anatomy and biochemistry of headache. Funct Neurol. 1993; 8(6):395–402.

[51] Buzzi MG. Trigeminal pain pathway: peripheral and central activation as experimental models of migraine. Funct Neurol. 2001; 16(4 Suppl):77–81.

[52] Evers S, Voss H, Bauer B, Sörös P, Husstedt IW. Peripheral autonomic potentials in primary headache and drug-induced headache. Cephalalgia. 1998; 18(4):216–221.

[53] Peroutka SJ. Migraine: a chronic sympathetic nervous system disorder. Headache. 2004; 44(1):53–64. doi: 10.1111/j.1526-4610.2004.04011.x

[54] Anthony M. Biochemical indices of sympathetic activity in migraine. Cephalalgia. 1981; 1(2):83–89.

[55] Sliwka U, Harscher S, Diehl RR, Van Schayck R, Niesen WD, Weiller C. Spontaneous oscillations in cerebral blood flow velocity give evidence of different autonomic dysfunctions in various types of headache. Headache. 2001; 41:157–163.

[56] Mamontov OV, Babayan L, Amelin AV, Giniatullin R, Kamshilin AA. Autonomous control of cardiovascular reactivity in patients with episodic and chronic forms of migraine. J Headache Pain. 2016; 17:52. doi: 10.1186/s10194-016-0645-6

[57] Shechter A, Stewart WF, Silberstein SD, Lipton RB. Migraine and autonomic nervous system function: a population-based, case-control study. Neurology. 2002; 58(3):422–427.

[58] Arbab MA, Wiklund L, Delgado T, Svendgaard NA. Stellate ganglion innervation of the vertebro-basilar arterial system demonstrated in the rat with anterograde and retrograde WGA-HRP tracing. Brain Res. 1988; 445:175–180.

[59] Edvinsson L, Uddman R. Neurobiology in primary headaches. Brain Res Brain Res Rev. 2005; 48(3):438-456.

[60] Edvinsson L, Goadsby PJ. Neuropeptides in migraine and cluster headache. Cephalalgia. 1994; 14(5):320–327.

[61] Edvinsson L, Uddman R. Adrenergic, cholinergic and peptidergic nerve fibres in dura mater- involvement in headache? Cephalalgia. 1981; 1(4):175–179. doi: 10.1016/j.brainresrev.2004.09.007

[62] Bjorklund H, Hokfelt T, Goldstein M, Terenius L, Olson L. Appearance of the noradrenergic markers tyrosine hydroxylase and neuropeptide Y in cholinergic nerves of the iris following sympathectomy. J Neurosci. 1985; 5:1633–1640.

[63] Gallai V, Sarchielli P, Trequattrini A, Paciaroni M, Usai F, Palumbo R. Neuropeptide Y in juvenile migraine and tension-type headache. Headache. 1994; 34(1):35–40.

[64] Lundberg JM, Rudehill A, Sollevi A, Theodorsson-Norheim E, Hamberger B. Frequency- and reserpine-dependent chemical coding of sympathetic transmission: differential release of noradrenaline and neuropeptide Y from pig spleen. Neurosci Lett. 1986; 63:96–100.

[65] Owman C, Edvinsson L. Histochemical and pharmacological approach to the investigation of neurotransmitters, with particular regard to the cerebrovascular bed. Ciba Found Symp. 1978; (56):275–311.

[66] Duverger D, Edvinsson L, MacKenzie ET, Oblin A, Rouquier L, Scatton B, Zivkovic B. Concentrations of putative neurovascular transmitters in major cerebral arteries and small pial vessels of various species. J Cereb Blood Flow Metab. 1987; 7(4):497–501.

[67] Rosendorff C, Mitchell G, Scriven DR, Shapiro C. Evidence for a dual innervation affecting local blood flow in the hypothalamus of the conscious rabbit. Circ Res. 1976; 38(3):140–145.

[68] Purkayastha S, Raven PB. The functional role of the alpha-1 adrenergic receptors in cerebral blood flow regulation. Indian J Pharmacol. 2011; 43(5):502–506. doi: 10.4103/0253-7613.84950.

[69] Suzuki N, Hardebo JE, Owman C. Origins and pathways of choline acetyltransferase-positive parasympathetic nerve fibers to cerebral vessels in rat. J Cereb Blood Flow Metab. 1990; 10:399–408.

[70] Hara H, Hamill GS, Jacobowitz DM. Origin of cholinergic nerves to the rat major cerebral arteries: coexistence with vasoactive intestinal polypeptide. Brain Res Bull. 1985; 14:179–188.

[71] Edvinsson L, Owman C, Sjoberg NO. Autonomic nerves, mast cells, and amine receptors in human brain vessels. A histochemical and pharmacological study. Brain Res. 1976; 115:377–393.

[72] Goadsby PJ, Edvinsson L, Ekman R. Release of vasoactive peptides in the extracerebral circulation of humans and the cat during activation of the trigeminovascular system. Ann Neurol. 1988; 23:193–196.

[73] Pietrobon D, Striessnig J. Neurobiology of migraine. Nat Rev Neurosci. 2003; 4(5):386–98.

[74] May A, Bahra A, Büchel C, Frackowiak RS, Goadsby PJ. PET and MRA findings in cluster headache and MRA in experimental pain. Neurology. 2000; 55(9):1328–1335.

[75] Goadsby PJ, Edvinsson L. The trigeminovascular system and migraine: studies characterizing cerebrovascular and neuropeptide changes seen in humans and cats. Ann Neurol. 1993; 33(1):48–56.

[76] Goadsby PJ, Uddman R, Edvinsson L. Cerebral vasodilatation in the cat involves nitric oxide from parasympathetic nerves. Brain Res. 1996; 707(1):110–8.

[77] Jansen-Olesen I, Goadsby PJ, Uddman R, Edvinsson L. Vasoactive intestinal peptide (VIP) like peptides in the cerebral circulation of the cat. J Auton Nerv Syst. 1994; 49 (Suppl):S97–103.

[78] Akerman S, Holland PR, Goadsby PJ. Diencephalic and brainstem mechanisms in migraine. Nat Rev Neurosci. 2011; 12:570–584. doi: 10.1038/nrn305

[79] Edvinsson L, Jansen I, Cunha e Sa M, Gulbenkian S. Demonstration of neuropeptide containing nerves and vasomotor responses to perivascular peptides in human cerebral arteries. Cephalalgia. 1994; 14:88–96.

[80] Amin FM, Hougaard A, Schytz HW, Asghar MS, Lundholm E, Parvaiz AI, de Koning PJ, Andersen MR, Larsson HB, Fahrenkrug J, Olesen J, Ashina M. Investigation of the

pathophysiological mechanisms of migraine attacks induced by pituitary adenylate cyclase-activating polypeptide-38. Brain. 2014; 137(Pt 3):779–794. doi: 10.1093/brain/awt369

[81] Møller Hansen J, Levy D. Pathophysiology of migraine: current status and future directions. In: Pathophysiology of Headaches Headache (Ashina M, Geppetti P, eds.), Springer International Publishing, Switzerland, 2015; pp. 212–229. doi: 10.1007/978-3-319-15621-7_12

[82] Takeshima T, Takao Y, Takahashi K. Pupillary sympathetic hypofunction and asymmetry in muscle contraction headache and migraine. Cephalagia. 1987; 7:257–262.

[83] Gotoh F, Komatsumoto S, Araki N, Gomi S. Noradrenergic nervous activity in migraine. Arch Neurol. 1984; 41(9):951–955.

[84] Rauschel V, Straube A, Süß F, Ruscheweyh R. Responsiveness of the autonomic nervous system during paced breathing and mental stress in migraine patients. J Headache Pain. 2015; 16:82. doi: 10.1186/s10194-015-0567-8

[85] Ashina M. Neurobiology of chronic tension-type headache. Cephalalgia. 2004;24(3): 161–72.

[86] Herman P. The pupil and headaches. Headache. 1983; 23:102–105.

[87] Yerdelen D, Acil T, Goksel B, Karatas M. Heart rate recovery in migraine and tension-type headache. Headache. 2008; 48(2):221–225. doi: 10.1111/j.1526-4610.2007.00994.x

[88] Tabata M, Takeshima T, Burioka N, Nomura T, Ishizaki K, Mori N, Kowa H, Nakashima K. Cosinor analysis of heart rate variability in ambulatory migraineurs. Headache. 2000; 40(6):457–463.

[89] Yildiz SK, Yildiz N, Korkmaz B, Altunrende B, Gezici AR, Alkoy S. Sympathetic skin responses from frontal region in migraine headache: a pilot study. Cephalalgia. 2008; 28(7):696–704. doi: 10.1111/j.1468-2982.2008.01574.x.

[90] Bugdayci G, Yildiz S, Altunrende B, Yildiz N, Alkoy S. Salivary alpha amylase activity in migraine patients. Auton Neurosci. 2010; 155(1–2):121–124. doi: 10.1016/j.autneu.2010.01.011

[91] Gass JJ, Glaros AG. Autonomic dysregulation in headache patients. Appl Psychophysiol Biofeedback. 2013; 38(4):257–263. doi: 10.1007/s10484-013-9231-8

[92] Tomé-Pires C, Miró J. Electrodermal responses and memory recall in migraineurs and headache-free controls. Eur J Pain. 2014; 18(9):1298–1306. doi:10.1002/j.1532-2149.2014.490.x.

[93] Costa A, Antonaci F, Ramusino MC, Nappi G. The neuropharmacology of cluster headache and other trigeminal autonomic cephalalgias. Curr Neuropharmacol. 2015; 13(3):304–323.

[94] Gottselig R, Messlinger K. Noxious chemical stimulation of rat facial mucosa increases intracranial blood flow through a trigemino-parasympathetic reflex-an experimental model for vascular dysfunctions in cluster headache. Cephalalgia. 2004; 24(3):206–214.

[95] Akerman S, Holland PR, Lasalandra MP, Goadsby PJ. Oxygen inhibits neuronal activation in the trigeminocervical complex after stimulation of trigeminal autonomic reflex, but not during direct dural activation of trigeminal afferents. Headache. 2009; 49(8):1131–1143. doi: 10.1111/j.1526-4610.2009.01501.x

[96] Dodick DW, Capobianco DJ. Treatment and management of cluster headache. Curr Pain Headache Rep. 2001; 5(1):83–91.

[97] Leistad RB, Sand T, Nilsen KB, Westgaard RH, Stovner LJ. Cardiovascular responses to cognitive stress in patients with migraine and tension-type headache. BMC Neurol. 2007; 7:23. doi: 10.1186/1471-2377-7-23

[98] Drew RC, Sinoway L. Autonomic Control of the Heart. In: Primer on the Autonomic Nervous System, Third Edition (Robertson D, Biaggioni I, Burnstock G, Low PA, Paton JFR, eds.), Academic Press, 2012: pp. 177–180. ISBN: 978-0-12-386525-0

[99] Porges SW. The polyvagal perspective. Biol Psychol. 2007; 74(2):116–143. DOI:10.1016/j.biopsycho.2006.06.009

[100] Dampney RA. Functional organization of central pathways regulating the cardiovascular system. Physiol Rev. 1994; 74:323–364.

[101] Taylor EW, Jordan D, Coote JH. Central control of the cardiovascular and respiratory systems and their interactions in vertebrates. Physiol Rev. 1999; 79(3):855–916.

[102] Benarroch EE. The central autonomic network: functional organization, dysfunction, and perspective. Mayo Clin Proc. 1993; 68(10):988–1001.

[103] Jones SE. Imaging for autonomic dysfunction. Cleve Clin J Med. 2011; 78(Suppl 1):S69–S74. doi: 10.3949/ccjm.78.s1.12

[104] Thayer JF, Hansen AL, Saus-Rose E, Johnsen BH. Heart rate variability, prefrontal neural function, and cognitive performance: the neurovisceral integration perspective on self-regulation, adaptation, and health. Ann Behav Med. 2009; 37(2):141–153. doi: 10.1007/s12160-009-9101-z

[105] Task force of the European Society of Cardiology and the North American Society of Pacing and Electrophysiology, Heart Rate Variability—standards of measurement, physiological interpretation and clinical use. Eur Heart J. 1996; 17:354–381. PMID: 8737210

[106] Salinger J, Pumprla J, Vychodil R, Stejskal P, Opavsky J, Novotny J, Bula J. Microcomputer system for telemetric assessment of short term heart rate variability in time and frequency domain, type VariaCardio TF4. Computers in Cardiology, IEEE. 1999;26:599–602.

[107] Taylor JA, Carr DL, Myers ChW, Eckberg DL. Mechanisms underlying very-low-frequency RR-interval oscillations in humans. Circulation. 1998; 98:547–555.

[108] Pogacnik T, Sega S, Pecnik B, Kiauta T. Autonomic function testing in patients with migraine. Headache. 1993; 33(10):545–50.

[109] Thomsen LL, Iversen HK, Boesen F, Olesen J. Transcranial Doppler and cardiovascular responses during cardiovascular autonomic tests in migraineurs during and outside attacks. Brain. 1995; 118:1319–1327.

[110] Benjelloun H, Birouk N, Slaoui I, Coghlan L. Autonomic profile of patients with migraine. Neuro Physiol Clin. 2005; 35(4):127–134.

[111] Havanka-Kanniainen H, Tolonen U, Myllyla VV. Autonomic dysfunction in adult migraineurs. Headache. 1986; 26:425–430.

[112] Martín R, Ribera C, Moltò JM, Ruiz C, Galiano L, Matías-Guiu J. Cardiovascular reflexes in patients with vascular headache. Cephalalgia. 1992; 12(6):360–4.

[113] Appel S, Kuritzky A, Zahavi I, Zigelman M, Akselrod S. Evidence for instability of the autonomic nervous system in patients with migraine headache. Headache. 1992; 32(1): 10–7.

[114] Matei D, Constantinescu V, Corciova C, Ignat B, Matei R, Popescu CD. Autonomic impairment in patients with migraine. Eur Rev Med Pharmacol Sci. 2015; 19(20):3922–7.

[115] Guinjoan SM, Castro MN, Vigo DE, Weidema H, Berbara C, Fahrer RD, et al. Depressive symptoms are related to decreased low-frequency heart rate variability in older adults with decompensated heart failure. Neuropsychobiology. 2007; 55(3–4):219–224. doi: 10.1159/000108381

[116] Lucini D, Di Fede G, Parati G, Pagani M. Impact of chronic psychosocial stress on autonomic cardiovascular regulation in otherwise healthy subjects. Hypertension. 2005; 46(5):1201–1206. doi:10.1161/01.HYP.0000185147.32385.4b

[117] Britton A, Malik M, Marmot M. The cardioprotective effects of alcohol consumption: does cardiac autonomic function play a role. Eur J Epidemiol. 2008; 23(2):105–108. doi: 10.1007/s10654-007-9213-3.

[118] Nater UM, Rohleder N.Salivary alpha-amylase as a non-invasive biomarker for the sympathetic nervous system: current state of research. Psychoneuroendocrinology. 2009; 34(4):486–496. doi: 10.1016/j.psyneuen.2009.01.014

[119] Romanowicz M, Schmidt JE, Bostwick JM, Mrazek DA, Karpyak VM. Changes in heart rate variability associated with acute alcohol consumption: current knowledge and implications for practice and research. Alcohol Clin Exp Res. 2011; 35(6):1092–1105. doi: 10.1111/j.1530-0277.2011.01442.x

[120] Barutcu I, Esen AM, Kaya D, Turkmen M, Karakaya O, Melek M, Esen OB, Basaran Y. Cigarette smoking and heart rate variability: dynamic influence of parasympathetic

and sympathetic maneuvers. Ann Noninvasive Electrocardiol. 2005; 10:324–329. doi: 10.1111/j.1542-474X.2005.00636.x

[121] Bonnemeier H, Richardt G, Potratz J, Wiegand UK, Brandes A, Kluge N, Katus HA. Circadian profile of cardiac autonomic nervous modulation in healthy subjects: differing effects of aging and gender on heart rate variability. J Cardiovasc Electrophysiol. 2003; 14(8):791–799. PMID: 12890036

[122] Berntson GG, Cacioppo JT, Grossman P. Whither vagal tone. Biol Psychol. 2007; 74(2): 295–300. doi: 10.1016/j.biopsycho.2006.08.006

[123] Lai TH, Fuh JL, Wang SJ. Cranial autonomic symptoms in migraine: characteristics and comparison with cluster headache. J Neurol Neurosurg Psychiatry. 2009; 80(10):1116–1119. doi: 10.1136/jnnp.2008.157743

[124] Hadjikhani N, Ward N, Boshyan J, Napodow V, Maeda Y, Truini A, Caramia F, Tinelli E, Mainero C. The missing link: enhanced functional connectivity between amygdala and visceroceptive cortex in migraine. Cephalalgia. 2013; 33:1264–1268.

[125] Perogamvros L, Schwartz S. The roles of the reward system in sleep and dreaming. Neurosci Biobehav Rev. 2012; 36:1934–1951.

[126] Ziegler DK, Hassanein RS, Kodanaz A, Meek JC. Circadian rhythms of plasma cortisol in migraine. J Neurol Neurosurg Psychiatry. 1979; 42(8):741–748. PMID: 573780

[127] van Hilten JJ, Ferrari MD, Van der Meer JW, Gijsman HJ, Looij BJ Jr. Plasma interleukin-1, tumour necrosis factor and hypothalamic-pituitary-adrenal axis responses during migraine attacks. Cephalalgia. 1991; 11(2):65–67.

[128] Dias-Ferreira E, Sousa JC, Melo I, Morgado P, Mesquita AR, Cerqueira JJ, Costa RM, Sousa N. Chronic stress causes frontostriatal reorganization and affects decision-making. Science. 2009; 325(5940):621–625.

[129] Kubera M, Obuchowicz E, Goehler L, Brzeszcz J, Maes M. In animal models, psychosocial stress-induced (neuro)inflammation, apoptosis and reduced neurogenesis are associated to the onset of depression. Prog Neuropsychopharmacol Biol Psychiatry. 2011; 35(3):744–59.

[130] Valfrè W, Rainero I, Bergui M, Pinessi L. Voxel-based morphometry reveals gray matter abnormalities in migraine. Headache. 2008; 48(1):109–17.

[131] Casucci G, Villani V, Finocchi C. Therapeutic strategies in migraine patients with mood and anxiety disorders: physiopathological basis. Neurol Sci. 2010; 31(Suppl 1):S99–S101.

[132] Peres MF, Sanchez del Rio M, Seabra ML, Tufik S, Abucham J, Cipolla-Neto J, Silberstein SD, Zukerman E. Hypothalamic involvement in chronic migraine. J Neurol Neurosurg Psychiatry. 2001; 71:747–751.

[133] McEwen BS. Sleep deprivation as a neurobiologic and physiologic stressor: allostasis and allostatic load. Metabolism. 2006b; 55(10, Suppl 2):S20–S23.

[134] Calhoun AH, Hutchinson S. Hormonal therapies for menstrual migraine. Curr Pain Headache Rep. 2009; 13:381–385.

[135] Borsook D, Maleki N, Becerra L, McEwen B. Understanding migraine through the lens of maladaptive stress responses: a model disease of allostatic load. Neuron. 2012; 73:219–234. doi: 10.1016/j.neuron.2012.01.001

[136] Goadsby PJ, Lipton RB. A review of paroxysmal hemicranias, SUNCT syndrome and other short-lasting headaches with autonomic feature, including new cases. Brain. 1997; 120(Pt 1):193–209.

[137] Goadsby PJ, Grosberg BM, Mauskop A, Cady R, Simmons KA. Effect of noninvasive vagus nerve stimulation on acute migraine: an open-label pilot study. Cephalalgia Int J Headache. 2014; 34(12):986–993. doi: 10.1177/0333102414524494]

[138] Lenaerts ME, Oommen KJ, Couch JR, Skaggs V. Can vagus nerve stimulation help migraine. Cephalalgia. 2008; 28:392–395. doi: 10.1111/j.1468-2982.2008.01538.x

[139] Cecchini AP, Mea E, Tullo V, Curone M, Franzini A, Broggi G, et al. Vagus nerve stimulation in drug-resistant daily chronic migraine with depression: preliminary data. Neurol Sci. 2009; 30(Suppl 1):S101–S104. doi: 10.1007/s10072-009-0073-3

[140] Nesbitt AD, Marin JCA, Tompkins E, Ruttledge MH, Goadsby PJ. Initial experience with a novel non-invasive vagus nerve stimulation device for the treatment of cluster headache. Neurology (Minneap). 2015; 84:1–5. doi: 10.1212/WNL.0000000000001394

[141] Leone M. Deep brain stimulation in headache. Lancet Neurol. 2006; 5(10):873–877. doi: 10.1016/S1474-4422(06)70575-0

[142] Leone M, May A, Franzini A, Broggi G, Dodick D, Rapoport A, Goadsby PJ, Schoenen J, Bonavita V, Bussone G. Deep brain stimulation for intractable chronic cluster headache: proposals for patient selection. Cephalalgia. 2004; 24(11):934–937. doi: 10.1111/j.1468-2982.2004.00742.x

[143] Schuh-Hofer S, Richter M, Geworski L, Villringer A, Israel H, Wenzel R, Munz DL, Arnold G. Increased serotonin transporter availability in the brainstem of migraineurs. J Neurol. 2007; 254(6):789–796. Epub 2007 Mar 12. doi: 10.1007/s00415-006-0444-0

[144] Mathew NT, Landy S, Stark S, Tietjen GE, Derosier FJ, White J, Lener SE, Bukenya D. Fixed-dose sumatriptan and naproxen in poor responders to triptans with a short half-life. Headache. 2009; 49(7):971–982. doi: 10.1111/j.1526-4610.2009.01458.x

[145] Dodick DW, Goadsby PJ, Spierings EL, Scherer JC, Sweeney SP, Grayzel DS. Safety and efficacy of LY2951742, a monoclonal antibody to calcitonin gene-related peptide, for the prevention of migraine: a phase 2, randomised, double-blind, placebo-controlled study. Lancet Neurol. 2014; 13(9):885–892. doi: 10.1016/S1474-4422(14)70128-0

[146] Schytz HW, Olesen J, Ashina M. The PACAP receptor: a novel target for migraine treatment. Neurotherapeutics. 2010 Apr; 7(2):191–196. doi: 10.1016/j.nurt.2010.02.003

[147] Holland P, Goadsby PJ. The hypothalamic orexinergic system: pain and primary headaches. Headache. 2007; 47(6):951–962. doi: 10.1111/j.1526-4610.2007.00842.x

[148] Jackson JL, Kuriyama A, Hayashino Y. Botulinum toxin A for prophylactic treatment of migraine and tension headaches in adults: a meta-analysis. JAMA. 2012; 307(16): 1736–1745. doi: 10.1001/jama.2012.505

[149] Rainero I, Rubino E, Paemeleire K, Gai A, Vacca A, De Martino P, Pinessi L. Genes and primary headaches: discovering new potential therapeutic targets. J Headache Pain. 2013; 14(1):61. http://DOI.org/10.1186/1129-2377-14-61

[150] Holroyd KA, Cottrell CK, O'Donnell FJ, Cordingley GE, Drew JB, Carlson BW, Himawan L. Effect of preventive (beta blocker) treatment, behavioural migraine management, or their combination on outcomes of optimised acute treatment in frequent migraine: randomised controlled trial. BMJ. 2010 Sep 29; 341:c4871. doi: 10.1136/bmj.c4871

Chapter 4

Relation between Smartphone Use and Unilateral Ocular Pain and Headache

Sertaç Argun Kıvanç, Berna Akova Budak,
Mahmut Oğuz Ulusoy, Osman Okan Olcaysü and
Nilüfer Yeşilırmak

Additional information is available at the end of the chapter

http://dx.doi.org/10.5772/66624

Abstract

Ocular pain and headache may stem from many causes, ranging from infections and inflammations to radiating pain. Nowadays, use of smartphones may be an emerging cause of unilateral ocular pain and headache, especially in young population. In this study, we implemented a survey and examined the eyes of patients who used smartphones with 20/20 vision. The patients with normal neurologic and ear-nose-throat (ENT) examination findings comprised the study group. The age, duration of smartphone use, ocular examination findings, and results of ocular surface disease index (OSDI) were recorded. An association between smartphone use and ocular pain/headache was found. Spherical equivalent values of the patients with headache or ocular pain were significantly lower than those who had no pain. The OSDI scores of patients with ocular pain were significantly higher than others without ocular pain. Adverse effects of smartphone use on ocular surface and over accommodation induced by near vision may have an effect on the occurrence of ocular pain and headache.

Keywords: accommodation, headache, ocular pain, ocular surface, smartphone

1. Introduction

Nowadays, smartphones are being used for a considerable time in daily life. Since these phones have the capability of performing many office tasks, they are increasingly used day by day. Although their smartphone use throughout the day makes life easier, they may lead to joint, posture, and some neurologic disorders [1, 2]. The most vulnerable organ during smartphone use is eyes. However, there is not much information about the effect of smartphones on eye in literature.

Eyes are organs that are in a way extension of the brain. Light rays entering the eye are transformed into chemical message by the specialized cells; rods and cones, and then ganglion cells are excited. This is mediated by bipolar cells. The bodies of ganglion cells are present in the retina, and the axons of these cells form the retinal nerve fiber layer and constitute optic nerve. The optic nerve exits the eyeball and course in the orbita, passes through the optic canal in the lesser wing of the sphenoid, enters cranium synapsing at superior colliculus, and then extends to visual cortex [3].

As eyes are extension of the nervous system, ocular pain may coexist with headache or many causes of pain may result from eye itself or structures around the eye [4, 5]. Migraine hemicrania continua and tension headache also lead to facial and ocular pain [6]. In seek of common and overlooked and avoidable causes of ocular pain such as smartphone use, the characteristics of patients with unilateral headache and/or ocular pain who use smartphones are investigated in this study.

2. Smartphone users

2.1. Material and methods

Medical records of patients with 20/20 visual acuity in both eyes that used smartphone in second half of 2015 were reviewed retrospectively. The patients with normal neurologic and ENT examination findings were included in the study. Biomicroscopic examination was done, and patients who had undergone ocular surgeries were excluded. Ocular surface diseases index (OSDI) scores and duration of the smartphone use were noted. Normal and cycloplegic refractive values of the patients were noted as spherical equivalent. Spherical equivalent is defined as the sum of spheric value and half of the cylinderic value. OSDI scores were measured with a questionnaire (**Figure 1**). Statistical analysis was performed with SPSS 22.

2.2. Findings

Seventy patients with 20/20 visual acuity in both eyes who use smartphone were identified. Fourteen of these patients had ocular pain and headache. Three of 70 patients had only ocular pain, and four of 70 patients had only headache. The age, gender, duration of smartphone use, normal and cycloplegic spherical equivalent values, and OSDI scores of the patients were shown in **Table 1**.

Spherical equivalent values of the patients with headache or ocular pain were significantly lower than those who had no pain. The OSDI scores of patients with ocular pain were significantly higher than others without ocular pain. Duration of smartphone use was given in **Table 2**.

2.3. Association between smartphone use and headache and eye pain

The eye has many visual functions, such as far vision, near vision, stereopsis, contrast sensitivity function, binocular, and mono vision [8]. Light stimulates the retinal pigment epithelium

http://dx.doi.org/10.5772/66624

Ocular Surface Disease Index© (OSDI©)[2]

Ask your patients the following 12 questions, and circle the number in the box that best represents each answer. Then, fill in boxes A, B, C, D, and E according to the instructions beside each.

Have you experienced any of the following *during the last week?*	All of the time	Most of the time	Half of the time	Some of the time	None of the time
1. Eyes that are sensitive to light? . .	4	3	2	1	0
2. Eyes that feel gritty?	4	3	2	1	0
3. Painful or sore eyes?	4	3	2	1	0
4. Blurred vision?	4	3	2	1	0
5. Poor vision?	4	3	2	1	0

Subtotal score for answers 1 to 5 [ ]

Have problems with your eyes limited you in performing any of the following *during the last week?*	All of the time	Most of the time	Half of the time	Some of the time	None of the time	N/A
6. Reading?	4	3	2	1	0	N/A
7. Driving at night?	4	3	2	1	0	N/A
8. Working with a computer or bank machine (ATM)?	4	3	2	1	0	N/A
9. Watching TV?	4	3	2	1	0	N/A

Subtotal score for answers 6 to 9 [ ]

Have your eyes felt uncomfortable in any of the following situations *during the last week?*	All of the time	Most of the time	Half of the time	Some of the time	None of the time	N/A
10. Windy conditions?	4	3	2	1	0	N/A
11. Places or areas with low humidity (very dry)?	4	3	2	1	0	N/A
12. Areas that are air conditioned? . . .	4	3	2	1	0	N/A

Subtotal score for answers 10 to 12 [ ]

Add subtotals A, B, and C to obtain D (D = sum of scores for all questions answered) [ ]

Total number of questions answered (do not include questions answered N/A) [ ]

Figure 1. An example of ocular surface disease index questionnaire [7].

and photoreceptors. As a result, chemical reaction starts and bipolar cells and ganglion cells are excited. And this excitation is conducted to visual cortex by optic nerve and optic radiation. Optic nerve is arranged by axons of approximately 1.2 million ganglion cells and divided into four segments. The first part and the shortest part are the intraocular segment, which one is called the optic disc and visible in ophthalmoscopic examination (**Figure 2**).

	Headache			Eye pain		
	+	–	*P* value	+	–	*P* value
Age	37.4	37.6	0.873	36.6	37.8	0.890
Gender (m/fm)	6/12	22/30	0.817	5/12	23/30	0.522
Duration of smartphone use (hour/day)	4.3	3.7	0.527	3.9	3.9	0.746
SE OD	0.20	0.93	**0.012**	0.21	0.93	**0.003**
CSE OD	0.57	0.96	0.216	0.92	0.92	0.880
SE OS	0.22	0.97	**0.015**	0.30	0.93	**0.012**
CSE OS	0.57	1.14	0.182	1.09	1.03	0.775
OSDI	42.4	36.6	0.298	44.1	32.0	**0.042**

OD, right eye; OS: left eye; SE, spherical equivalent; CSE, cycloplegic spherical equivalent.
Note: Bold entries are **p<0.05**.

Table 1. The age, gender, duration of smartphone use, spherical equivalent values and OSDI scores of the patients.

The second part is intraorbital segment. The length of this part is about 0.2–0.3 cm long. This segment ends with optic foramen and myelin sheaths are added to the nerve fibers in this segment. The segment that traverses in the optic canal is called intracanalicular segment. This part is fixed to the canal, because dura mater fuses with the periosteum. Last part of the optic nerve is intracranial segment. This part joins the chiasm, and the length is about 10 mm [3]. After chiasm, the retro-chiasmal part of optic tract starts. Axons of ganglion cells make synapsis at lateral geniculate nucleus. After this point, optic radiations start and terminate at visual cortex. These connections simply provide the pathway for the normal vision. However, we need additional features for near vision. In an eye, especially young ones, three physiological responses occur when the eye tries to focus at near. These are accommodation, the pupil constriction, and the convergence of the eyes (accommodative triad). These three actions are coordinated by the preganglionic parasympathetic innervation from the Edinger-Westphal (EW) nucleus [6]. All of these pathways should function properly to use a smartphone, because usually people hold smartphones 30–35 cm far away from their eyes requiring healthy near reflex.

According to this study, it is likely that there is an association between smartphone use and ocular pain and headache. In the literature, there is scanty information related to this finding.

In the past, it was suggested that mobile phones may cause headache [8]. Also, blurring of vision was significantly increased in users of mobile phones who possessed mobile phone

		Headache	
		+	–
Eye pain	+	4.0 ± 1.9	3.8 ± 2.7
	–	5.0 ± 2.7	3.8 ± 2.3

Table 2. Duration of smartphone use.

http://dx.doi.org/10.5772/66624

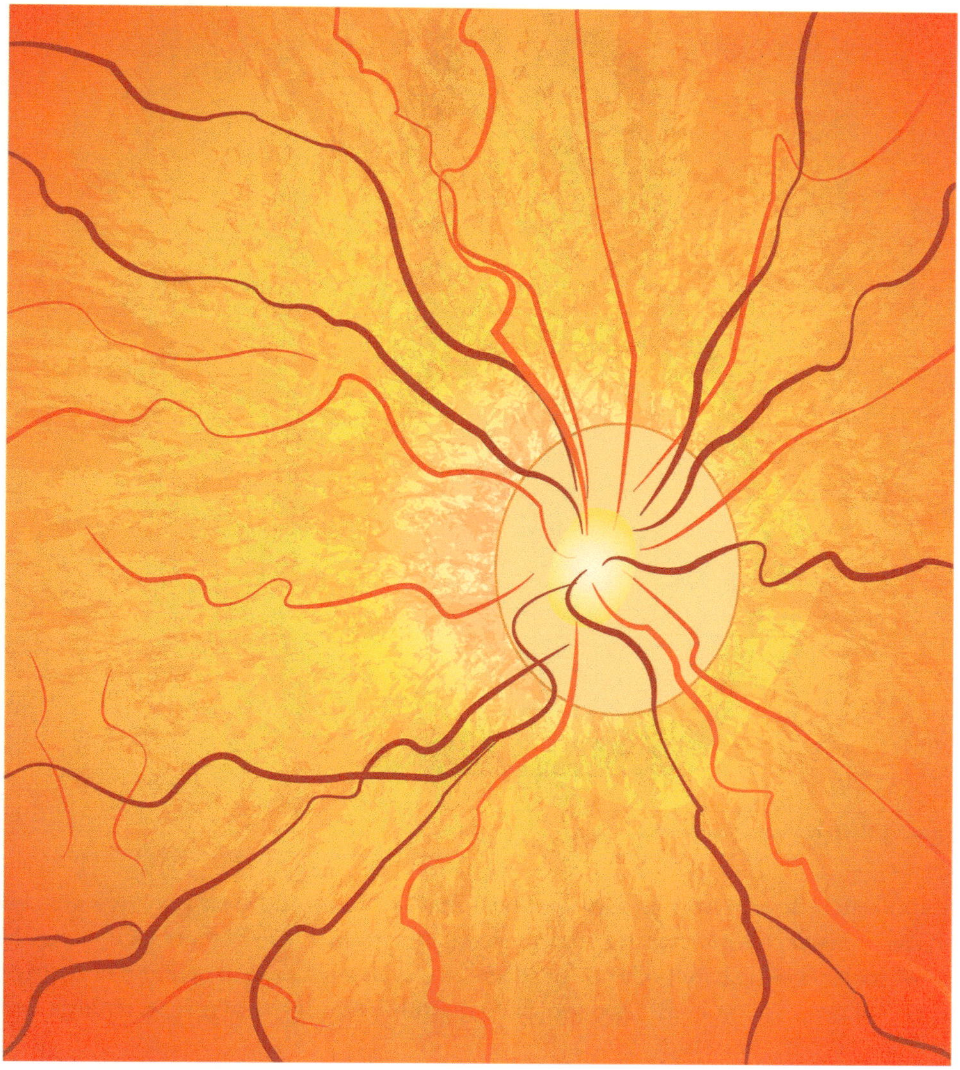

Figure 2. View of optic disc.

more than 2 years [9]. In a large population-based study which included 1025 subjects aged between 13 and 17 years, no consistent associations between the use of electronic media (mobile phones, computer, watching television, and playing with game consoles) and different types of headache were reported [10]. On the other hand, in another study, a significant association between increasing screen time (computers, smartphones, tablets, and television) exposure and migraine was found and no significant association was found with non-migraine headache in young adults [2]. In this study, no association was detected between duration of smartphone use and ocular pain or headache. However, the sample size of this study may be small to detect such a relation. We realized that when we use smartphone, we hold the phone in front of our dominant eye for near vision (**Figure 3**).

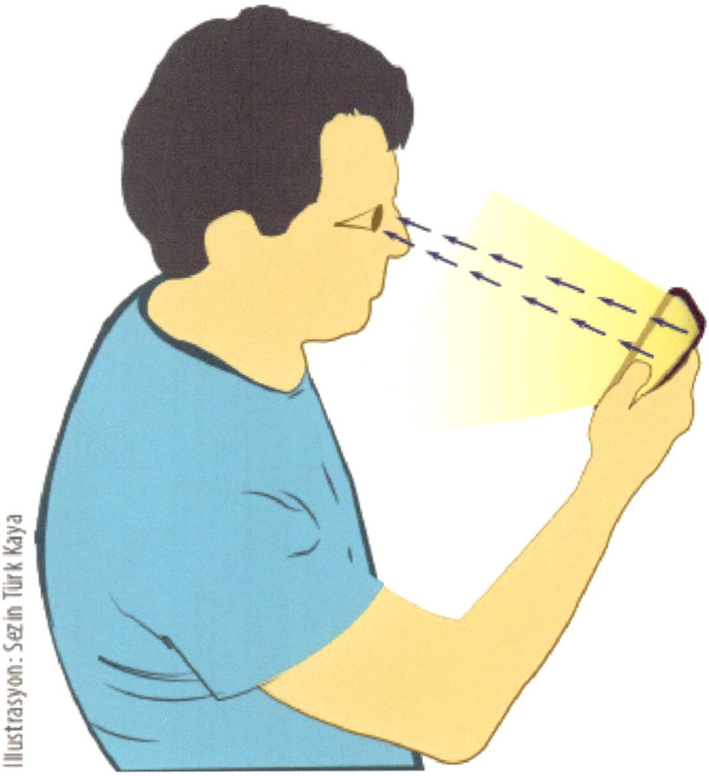

Figure 3. Subject holding smartphone.

We think that direct effect of light and heat that is produced by smartphone affects ocular surface. This effect is much more pronounced in the patient with higher OSDI scores. In other words, patients, who had moderate or severe dry eye, are at risks of ocular pain with overuse of smartphones. Moon et al. reported that smartphone usage is higher in children with dry eye diseases than controls [11].

In previous studies, it was shown that dry eye might cause corneal sensitivity and pain around eye [12]. However, this thesis does not explain why headache incidence is high in those patients. This may also be explained by over accommodation. It was mentioned previously that over accommodation is a cause of ocular pain [13]. In this study, spherical equivalent values of the patients with headache or ocular pain were significantly lower than those who had no pain, but the cycloplegic values were not different. The patients with ocular pain or headache accommodated more when compared to other smartphone users without pain. The refraction has also been studied in migraine patients with aura and without aura and controls, and lower cycloplegic values were identified in migraine patients with aura [14]. Adverse effects of smartphone use on ocular surface and over accommodation induced by near vision may have an effect on occurrence of ocular pain and headache. Further prospective studies with larger populations may clarify the association of smartphone use and ocular pain and headache.

Author details

Sertaç Argun Kıvanç[1], Berna Akova Budak[1]*, Mahmut Oğuz Ulusoy[2], Osman Okan Olcaysü[3] and Nilüfer Yeşilırmak[4]

*Address all correspondence to: bernaakova@hotmail.com

1 Department of Ophthalmology, School of Medicine, Uludag University, Bursa, Turkey

2 Department of Ophthalmology, Research Center, Başkent University, Konya, Turkey

3 Department of Ophthalmology, Erzurum Region Education and Training Hospital, Erzurum, Turkey

4 Department of Ophthalmology, Ankara Education and Region Hospital, University of Health Sciences, Ankara, Turkey

References

[1] Kim SY, Koo SJ. Effect of duration of smartphoneuse on muscle fatigue and pain caused by forward head posture in adults. J Phys Ther Sci. 2016;**28**:1669–72. doi:10.1589/jpts.28.1669

[2] Montagni I, Guichard E, Carpenet C, Tzourio C, Kurth T. Screen time exposure and reporting of headaches in young adults: a cross-sectional study. Cephalalgia. 2015; **36**:1020–1027.

[3] Bowling B, editor. Kanski's Clinical Ophthalmology. 8th ed. Oxford, Elsevier; 2015.

[4] Tomsak RL. Ophthalmologic aspects of headache. Med Clin North Am. 1991;**75**:693–706.

[5] Ringeisen AL, Harrison AR, Lee MS. Ocular and orbital pain for the headache specialist. Curr Neurol Neurosci Rep. 2011;**11**:156–63. doi:10.1007/s11910-010-0167-6

[6] Levin LA, Nilsson SFE, Ver Hoeve J, Wu SM, editors. Adler's Physiology of the Eye. 11th ed. Mosby, Oxford, Elsevier; 2011.

[7] Walt J, Rowe M, Stern K. Evaluating the functional impact of dry eye: the ocular surface disease index (Abstract). Drug Inf J. 1997;**31**:1436.

[8] Balikci K, Cem Ozcan I, Turgut-Balik D, Balik HH. A survey study on some neurological symptoms and sensations experienced by long term users of mobile phones. Pathol Biol (Paris). 2005;**53**:30–4.

[9] Küçer N. Some ocular symptoms experienced by users of mobile phones. Electromagn Biol Med. 2008;**27**:205–9. doi:10.1080/15368370802072174

[10] Milde-Busch A, vonKries R, Thomas S, Heinrich S, Straube A, Radon K. The association between use of electronic media and prevalence of headache inadolescents: results from a population-based cross-sectional study. BMC Neurol. 2010;**10**:12. doi:10.1186/1471-237 7-10-12

[11] Moon JH, Lee MY, Moon NJ. Association between video display terminal use and dry eye disease in school children. J Pediatr Ophthalmol Strabismus. 2014;**51**:87–92. doi:10.3928/01913913-20140128-01

[12] Kaido M, Kawashima M, Ishida R, Tsubota K. Relationship of corneal pain sensitivity with dry eye symptoms in dry eye with short tear break-up time. Invest Ophthalmol Vis Sci. 2016;**57**:914–9. doi:10.1167/iovs.15-18447

[13] Sterner B, Gellerstedt M, Sjöström A. Accommodation and the relationship to subjective symptoms with near work for young school children. Ophthalmic Physiol Opt. 2006;**26**:148–55.

[14] Kıvanç SA, Ulusoy MO, Akova-Budak B, Olcaysu OO, Özcan ME. Is ciliary muscle affected in migraine patients with aura and without aura? Med Sci Monit. 2015;**21**:1214–8. doi:10.12659/MSM.893307

Chapter 5

Trichodynia (Scalp Dysesthesia)

Müge Güler Özden

Additional information is available at the end of the chapter

http://dx.doi.org/10.5772/67792

Abstract

Trichodynia is defined as a painful sensation in the skin of the scalp or the hair without an underlying cutaneous disease. The term "trichodynia" (cutaneous dysesthesia syndrome) has also been proposed for discomfort, pain, burning, or stinging of the scalp related to diffuse alopecia. Probably, the diffuse alopecia or telogen effluvium and trichodynia are related. The underlying mechanisms creating the pain are not clear, though it has been proposed that it is probably multi-etiological. The most accepted hypotheses are increased expression of the neuropeptide substance P, underlying psychiatric disorders, nutritional deficiencies, and perifollicular inflammation. Although dealing with trichodynia can be distressing and literature support is weak, there are a number of treatments available.

Keywords: trichodynia, scalp pain, scalp dysesthesia, cutaneous dysesthesia syndrome

1. Introduction

Trichodynia is defined as a painful sensation in the skin of the scalp or the hair itself and becomes more intense when hairs are touched. Before making a diagnosis of "trichodynia," the physician must be sure that there is no cutaneous disease [1]. If the patient reports headache or temporal pain by palpation, tension headaches or temporal arteritis should be evaluated first. The term "trichodynia" (cutaneous dysesthesia syndrome) has also been proposed for discomfort, pain, burning, or stinging of the scalp related to diffuse alopecia. It has been found that 34% of female patients with hair loss complained of this phenomenon [2]. In a recent survey, Grimalt et al. showed that 14% of their diffuse alopecia patients reported trichodynia [3]. Complaints such as pain and burning of the scalp in patients with diffuse alopecia were described in the earlier dermatology literature [2, 4]. Both such studies and clinical observations have led to the idea that the diffuse alopecia or telogen effluvium (TE) and trichodynia are related. By definition, TE is a nonscarring and diffuse hair loss from the scalp that occurs a few months after a triggering event.

2. Ethiopathology

The underlying mechanisms creating the pain are not clear, though it has been proposed that it is probably multi-etiological. The most accepted hypotheses are increased expression of the neuropeptide substance P (SP), underlying psychiatric disorders, nutritional deficiencies, and perifollicular inflammation [1, 2, 5–7]. Substance P is involved in pain perception by the nerve endings, and changes in the production and activity of substance P around the hair follicles may be responsible for the pain and burning sensation [8]. Hair follicles are innervated by unmyelinated neural plexuses located around the hair follicle stem cells. These nerve fibers contain neuropeptides including substance P (SP) and calcitonin gene-related peptide (CGRP). These neuropeptides play an important role in the regulation of hair growth and are associated with the neurogenic inflammatory response. Perifollicular SP is also involved in the regulation of hair growth [9]. An imbalance in the tonic release of neuropeptides may result in inhibition of hair growth. Cutrer et al. hypothesized that chronic activation of the c-fibers, in addition to mediating inflammatory pain and follicular injury, might reduce SP and CGRP concentrations resulting in altered peribulbar antigen presentation and inhibition of further hair growth [10].

Another explanation may be an underlying psychiatric disorder. It has been found that 76% of the people who had trichodynia had psychopathic signs versus 20% in the control group, supporting this idea. Researchers have observed and speculated that there is a connection between psychopathologic findings (such as anxiety) and trichodynia [1, 5, 6, 11–14]. In 2006 Gupta and Gupta. found that numbness and pain are common symptoms of somatoform dissociation or conversion reaction [15]. Kivanç et al. found that trichodynia was associated with depression in the telogen alopecia group and with obsessive-compulsive personality disorder in the androgenic alopecia group [16]. However, this idea is controversial. Although increased rates of psychiatric problems have been reported in patients with trichodynia, Ozturk et al. found no association between trichodynia and depression or anxiety [17]. In this study the patients with telogen alopecia were consisting the control group, and they could have the opportunity to evaluate only the trichodynia patients.

Neuropathic pain can also be associated with nutritional deficiencies (Fe, B12, ferritin, zinc, vitamin D, vitamin E). Nutritional factors affect the hair directly, and dietary supplements containing B complex vitamins can influence hair growth [17–19]. Nutritional deficiencies have been reported in other cutaneous dysesthesia syndromes. For example, glossodynia is characterized by a burning sensation of the tongue and oral mucosa. Menopause, psychogenic disorders, and nutritional factors have also been suggested to cause this phenomenon [13]. However, evidence level is very low to confirm this nutritional hypothesis for trichodynia patients [20].

3. Treatment

Trichodynia symptoms are of great relevance to patients and place the physician in a challenging diagnostic and therapeutic situation. Although dealing with trichodynia can be distressing and literature support is weak, there are a number of treatments available. L-Cystine-containing oral preparations, topical corticosteroids (both high potency and low), and anti-inflammatory drugs have been advocated (remember inflammatory hypothesis). Inhibitors of SP can also be tried. Cannabinoids, for example, have been demonstrated to inhibit SP [21]. Capsaicin cream has been used because it blocks substance P when applied to the hair follicles. On the basis of psychiatric origin, the physician also may use low-dose antidepressants (venlafaxine, amitriptyline, and doxepin) and also pregabalin [22, 23].

In 2009, Cutrer et al. have investigated the efficacy of botulinum toxin treatment in cephalalgia alopecia patients and obtained improved pain control and hair regrowth following BoNT/A injections [10]. They also observed that botulinum increases substance P and calcitonin gene-related peptide-containing cutaneous nerves in the scalp. BoNT/A does not block low-level trophic release of neuropeptides such as CGRP and allows resumption of SP and CGRP baseline regulation of the hair follicle and hair regrowth [24]. However, we should keep in mind that BoNT/A treatment is temporary. The process of painful inflammatory activation, hair follicle regression, and hair loss is repeated after a few months.

Sensory tests revealed that trichodynia patients were significantly more sensitive to touch and to pressure pain and exhibited cranial mechanical hyperesthesia and cranial hyperalgesia [25]. So, gentle scalp maintenance may provide some relief. To support the treatment, it is important to inform the patients about not to use over hot water and harsh shampoos or wear tight pony tail. Other relaxation techniques such as gentle scalp massage may also help in reducing symptoms.

4. Other dermatological conditions causing scalp pain

Scalp pain can occur with cicatricial alopecia that can be caused by a fungus infection or autoimmune conditions such as cutaneous lupus and lichen planopilaris. Folliculitis decalvans and dissecting cellulitis are forms of primary neutrophilic scarring alopecia that are characterized clinically by chronic suppurative folliculitis and often associated with pruritus or even pain. The inflammatory cells may irritate nerve endings leading to a burning or painful sensation. Hair dye-related dermatitis may also cause burning sensations.

There are also painful tumoral lesions of the skin and subcutaneous tissue. These lesions can be found anywhere in the peripheral nerve tissue. They have a propensity for developing on the skin and subcutaneous tissue, as well as in oral and pharyngeal locations. An old acronym may help us to remember them. LEND AN EGG tumors (leiomyoma, eccrine spiradenoma, neuroma, dermatofibroma, angiolipoma, neurilemmoma, endometrioma, glomus tumor, and granular cell tumors) must always be considered when there is a tumoral lesion associated with pain [26].

Author details

Müge Güler Özden

Address all correspondence to: mgulerozden@hotmail.com

Medical Faculty, Department of Dermatology, Ondokuz Mayıs University, Samsun, Turkey

References

[1] Willimann B, Trüeb RM. Hair pain (trichodynia): Frequency and relationship to hair loss and patient gender. Dermatology. 2002;205:374–7.

[2] Rebora A, Semino MT, Guarrera M. Trichodynia. Dermatology. 1996;192:292–3.

[3] Grimalt R, Ferrando J, Grimalt F. Trichodynia. Dermatology. 1998;196(3):374.

[4] Hoss D, Segal S. Scalp dysesthesia. Arch Dermatol. 1998;134:327–30.

[5] Trüeb RM. Telogen effluvium and trichodynia. Dermatology. 1998;96:374–5.

[6] Trüeb RM. Idiopathic chronic telogen effluvium in the woman. Hautarzt. 2000;51:899–905.

[7] Baldari M, Montinari M, Guarrera M, Rebora A. Trichodynia is a distinguishing symptom of telogen effluvium. J Eur Acad Dermatol Venereol. 2009;23:733–4.

[8] Ericson M, Gabrielson A, Worel S, Lee WS, Hordinsky MK. Substance P (SP) in innervated and non-innervated blood vessels in the skin of patients with symptomatic scalp. Exp Dermatol. 1999;8:344–5.

[9] Paus R, Heinzelmann T, Schultz KD, Furkert J, Fechner K, Czarnetzki BM. Hair growth induction by substance P. Lab Investig. 1994;71:134–40.

[10] Cutrer FM, Sandroni P and Wendelschafer-Crabb G. Botulinum toxin treatment of cephalalgia alopecia increases substance P and calcitonin gene-related peptide-containing cutaneous nerves in scalp. Cephalalgia. 2010;30(8):1000–6.

[11] Ericson M, Gabrielson A, Rief W, Hiller W, Geissner E, Fichter MM. A two-year follow-up study of patients with somatoform disorders. Psychosomatics. 1995;36:376–86.

[12] Buchanan JA, Zakrzewska JM. Burning mouth syndrome. Clin Evid (Online). 2010;19:1301.

[13] Moore PA, Guggenheimer J, Orchard T. Burning mouth syndrome and peripheral neuropathy in patients with type 1 diabetes mellitus. J Diabet Complicat. 2007;21:397–402.

[14] Durusoy C, Ozenli Y, Adiguzel A, Budakoglu IY, Tugal O, Arikan S, et al. The role of psychological factors and serum zinc, folate and vitamin B12 levels in the aetiology of trichodynia: A case-control study. Clin Exp Dermatol. 2009;34:789–92.

[15] Gupta MA, Gupta AK. Stressful major life events are associated with a higher frequency of cutaneous sensory symptoms: An empirical study of non-clinical subjects. J Eur Acad Dermatol Venereol. 2004;18:560–5.

[16] Kivanç-Altunay I, Savaş C, Gökdemir G, Köşlü A, Ayaydin EB. The presence of trichodynia in patients with telogen effluvium and androgenetic alopecia. Int J Dermatol. 2003;42:691–3.

[17] Ozturk P, Orhan FO, Ozer A, Akman Y, Kurutas E. Evaluation of anxiety and levels of serum B12, folate, TSH, ferritin, and zinc in telogen alopecia patients with trichodynia. Int J Trichol. 2012;4(4):251–4.

[18] Rushton DH. Nutritional factors and hair loss. Clin Exp Dermatol. 2002;27:396–404.

[19] Lengg N, Heidecker B, Seifert B, Trueb RM. Dietary supplement increases anagen hair rate in women with telogen effluvium: Results of double-blind, placebo-controlled trial. Therapy. 2007;4:59–65.

[20] Durusoy, Ozturk P, Orhan FO, Ozer A, Akman Y, Kurutas E. Evaluation of anxiety and levels of serum B12, folate, TSH, ferritin, and zinc in telogen alopecia patients with trichodynia. Int J Trichol. 2012;4(4):251–4.

[21] OConnor TM, OConnell J, Obrien DJ, et al. The role of substance P in inflammatory disease. J Cell Physiol. 2004;201:167–180.

[22] Sarifakioğlu E, Onur O. Women with scalp dysesthesia treated with pregabalin. Int J Dermatol. 2013;52:1398–1461.

[23] Thorsberry L, English J. Scalp dysesthesia related to cervical spine disease. JAMA Dermatol. 2013;149:200–3.

[24] Durham PL, Cady R, Cady R. Regulation of calcitonin gene-related peptide secretion from trigeminal nerve cells by botulinum toxin type A: Implications for migraine therapy. Headache. 2004;44:35–43.

[25] Defrin R, Lurie R. Indications for peripheral and central sensitization in patients with chronic scalp pain (trichodynia). Clin J Pain. 2001;29(5):417–424.

[26] Naversen DN, Trask DM, Watson FH, Burket JM. Painful tumors of the skin: "LEND AN EGG". J Am Acad Dermatol. 1993;28(2):298–300.

Section 2

Therapeutical Aspects in Headache

Chapter 6

Surgical Therapy of Migraine and Tension-Type Headache

Edoardo Raposio, Nicolò Bertozzi,
Chiara Bordin and Francesco Simonacci

Additional information is available at the end of the chapter

http://dx.doi.org/10.5772/64652

Abstract

During the last few years, multiple studies have demonstrated the efficacy of migraine and tension-type headache trigger site deactivation surgery, hence expanding the therapeutic potentiality of plastic surgery. These procedures are performed based on headache onset and location: four trigger points that may cause the compression of the trigeminal branches have been described. In the present chapter, we describe indications, contraindications, procedures, and results of this therapy, focusing on our approach that relies on one 1-cm incision, and it is performed under local anesthesia.

Keywords: migraine, tension-type headache, surgical therapy, endoscopic surgery, minimally invasive surgery

1. Introduction

Migraine headaches (MH) affect over 324.1 million people worldwide [1]. Despite its prevalence and debilitating nature, MH is still widely undiagnosed and undertreated. The direct and indirect cost due to MH treatment accounts for $13 to $17 billion each year only in the USA [2]. Every year 112 million workdays are missed because of MH, with a $14 billion annual loss of productivity in the USA [3]. MH has an even greater burden on patients' everyday life, their families, and the society.

Traditionally, MH has been managed with a combination of non-pharmacologic (behavioral) treatment and abortive or preventive drugs. Despite advancements in pharmaceutical therapies (the annual cost of medications alone is $1.5 billion), almost 30% of MH patients are refractory to standard treatment and still suffering from persistent MH. Furthermore, numerous side effects are reported in the literature as a consequence of chronic MH drugs use, such as fatigue; dizziness; cardiovascular arrhythmias; cerebral, myocardial, and peripheral ischemia; hypertension; and hepatotoxicity.

Over the years, various hypotheses have been proposed to reveal MH etiology. Researchers have attributed MH origin to central neurovascular phenomena, cortical neuronal hyperexcitability, cortical spreading depression, and abnormal modulation of brain nociceptive system; finally, central and peripheral activation with sensitization of the trigeminal system was casted as the main MH cause [4]. What is clear is that MH pathophysiology is still a matter of debate.

Plastic surgeons were not looking for a surgical treatment for MH; however, this idea made its way in 1999 following the report made by patients that described elimination or improvement in their MH after corrugator supercilii muscle resection for forehead rejuvenation surgery [4]. In 2000, Guyuron et al. first reported in a retrospective study this association between corrugator supercilii muscle resection and disappearance or significant improvement in MH attacks. In the same years, independent studies demonstrated the efficacy of botulin toxin injection for the treatment of MH [4].

These evidences supported the hypothesis that MH was determined by peripheral activation of the trigeminal nerve, due to overstimulation of its branches (trigger points), followed by peripheral and central sensitization [5]. The trigger site is defined as the point where the MH starts and corresponds to the anatomical area of potential irritation of the trigeminal nerve [5]. Consequence of the mechanical stimulation and irritation of the trigeminal nerve is the release of calcitonin gene-related peptide, substance P, and neurokinin, which are found in cell bodies of trigeminal nerves [4, 5]. These neuropeptides may cause the activation of the trigeminovascular system and the neurogenic inflammation that are followed by meningeal irritation, altered microvascular blood flow, central and peripheral trigeminal sensitization recognized as hyperalgesia, and cutaneous allodynia.

The hypothesis that compression of craniofacial nerves could play a key role in triggering migraines has been strengthened by multiple anatomical studies demonstrating that musculature, vessels, bony foramen, and fascial bands can entrap or compress nerve branches at proposed migraine trigger sites [5, 6].

Over the last 15 years, Guyuron conducted several studies providing foundation for this hypothesis and reported a reduction of the frequency, duration, and intensity of MH by at least half in 80–90% of patients [4, 6–8]. In the same years, other independent groups reported similar findings using Guyuron's protocols, demonstrating the effectiveness of the procedure and the reproducibility of the results [5]. However, the most striking evidence for the effectiveness of peripheral nerve decompression surgery for MH therapy is derived from a double-blind, sham-controlled study conducted by Guyuron [7]. In this trial, 49 patients underwent decompressive surgery, while 26 underwent sham surgery. At least 50% reduction in MH was reported from 57.7% of patients of the sham surgery group and 83.7% in the actual surgery group ($p = 0.05$). Moreover, 57.1% of actual surgical group reported complete elimination of

MH symptoms, compared with only 3.8% of patients in the sham surgery group ($p = 0.001$). At 1 year, all migraine headache measurements were significantly improved in the actual surgical group and were not dependent on the trigger site.

Research has established that deactivation surgery could be performed at four main trigger sites and two less common ones [9]:

1. Frontal trigger (Site I): patients with frontal symptoms; the glabellar muscles or vessels may irritate the supratrochlear and supraorbital nerves.

2. Temporal trigger (Site II): patients with temporal headaches; the temporalis muscle or vessels may cause inflammation of the zygomatic temporal branch of the trigeminal nerve.

3. Rhinogenic trigger (Site III): patients complain of paranasal and retrobulbar headaches; deviated septum, contact between the turbinates and the septum, concha bullosa, septa bullosa, and other intranasal abnormalities may irritate the trigeminal end branches. This site will not be covered in the present chapter.

4. Greater occipital trigger (Site IV): patients refer occipital symptoms: occipitalis, trapezius, and semispinalis capitis muscles, fascial bands, or the occipital artery can irritate the greater occipital nerve (GON).

5. Auriculotemporal trigger (Site V): patients complain of temporal headaches; in the preauricular and temple region, the superficial temporal artery and fascial bands may be the cause of auriculotemporal nerve irritation.

6. Lesser occipital trigger (Site VI): patients refer occipital symptoms; trapezius and sternocleidomastoid muscles, fascial bands, and occipital artery branches may compress the lesser occipital nerve.

Essential step is detecting the precise site of pain onset [10]. Although patients may report diffuse headache, once they are asked to locate where the pain begins, they can precisely identify it by pointing with one fingertip, and that is where the surgical treatment must be focused on to release the nerve branch involved. Surgeons can confirm the correct localization of the trigger point by simple compression on the tender point, which usually evoke pain. Nerve blocks and the use of a portable Doppler device could also confirm the trigger points and may help surgeons until they develop sufficient comfort and expertise, while preoperative botulinum toxin injections have proven to be useless. Lack or incomplete response should be carefully interpreted as does not automatically exclude the suspected trigger point. Thus, the analysis of patients' symptoms and the physical examination can reliably guide the surgical planning.

Therefore, the mechanism of surgical deactivation of MH trigger sites is similar to carpal tunnel surgery or other nerve decompression techniques. There are strong evidences that surgical treatment for MH can successfully eliminate or reduce the MH frequency, intensity, and duration in a lasting manner, reducing the economic burden of MH sufferers, improving patients' performances and participation in daily life activities [2, 9]. However there are still a percentage of patients that are refractory to surgery [6]. Possible explanation is the incomplete detection of all of the trigger sites or that the irritation sites were not correctly dealt by current surgical approaches [5]. Rigorous patient screening and selection and proper identification of MH trigger points are mandatory for successful surgical outcome; yet a thorough understanding of the anatomy is essential to ensure complete nerve release and prevent postoperative complications.

2. Surgical anatomy

2.1. Frontal region

The frontal region constitutes the upper third of the face. It is an unpaired and median anatomic region, which extends from the hair margin of the scalp to the eyebrows overlying the supraorbital rim. It consists of multiple tissue layers: there are the skin, which here is the thickest of the face, a subcutaneous layer of fibro-adipose tissue, and a myofascial layer. The myofascial portion lays on the periosteum of the frontalis bone [11].

The muscles of the frontal region can be divided into two groups regarding their function. For the elevators' group, there is the frontal belly of the occipitofrontalis, whose insertions to the deep layer of the skin are distributed from the aponeurotic galea to the brow level, where the superior arc of the periorbital septum provides an indirect bony origin [11]. The depressor group features the glabellar muscle group, including the procerus, the corrugator supercilii, the depressor supercilii, and the orbicularis oculi muscles. These muscles extend through the galeal fat pad before giving off their dermal insertions and are often blended with fibers of the frontalis muscle.

The procerus is a small, triangular muscle that originates from the fascia of the nasal bone and inserts into the glabellar and forehead skin. Superior to the procerus, there is the corrugator supercilii muscle, a small pyramidal muscle, which extends obliquely over the supraorbital rim. It has two heads, transverse and oblique. The first one is found from the nasal process of the frontal bone to the dermis at the middle third of the brow, while the second one is smaller and parallel to the fibers of the depressor supercilii. The depressor supercilii muscle arises from the medial orbital rim, near the lacrimal sac, and inserts on the medial aspect of the bony orbit, inferior to the corrugators supercilii. The orbicularis oculi is a flat elliptical muscle which surrounds the orbit and spreads in the adjacent regions of the eyelids, anterior temporal region, infraorbital cheek, and superciliary region. It divides in an orbital, preseptal, and pretarsal portion. The orbital portion arches around the orbit stemming from the nasal component of the frontal bone, from the frontal process of the maxilla, and from the medial canthal tendon. The preseptal or palpebral portion overlies the orbital septum with its fibers originating from the superficial surface of the medial canthal tendon and from the bone immediately above and below it and then converging at the lateral palpebral raphe. The pretarsal or lacrimal portion lies over the tarsus, and its fibers adhere to it following an elliptical path and laterally interlace with the lateral raphe. A number of ligamentous attachments are found in the frontal region stemming from the temporal ligamentous adhesion. It arises from the periosteum of the frontal bone, and it forms a triangular structure 20 mm high with a base of 15 mm situated 10 mm above the arcus marginalis of the rim and parallel to it. Three ligaments radiate from it: the superior and inferior temporal septum, belonging to the temple region, and the supraorbital adhesion. They are responsible of the compartmentation of the forehead and the brow together with the periorbital septum which divides the orbital region in the periorbital and orbital compartments.

The supraorbital ligamentous adhesion is located between the temporal ligament and the origin of the corrugator muscle. Its inferior border lies 6 mm above the deep attachment of the periorbital septum, while the upper border is not well defined and extends cranially a variable of 20–40 mm above the orbital rim.

The periorbital septum connects the inferomedial origin of the orbicularis oculi with that of corrugator muscle, occupying three-quarters of the orbital rim. In the periorbital portion, it continues as the fibrous periosteum, while the orbital region goes on to form the orbital septum. These structures avoid contributing to ocular complication as consequence of the surgical decompression of the nerves, since they are effective in isolating the edema in the forehead region and are dissected within the surgical decompression of the supraorbital and the supratrochlear nerves [4–6, 12].

The supraorbital nerve is a sensory nerve originating from the frontal branch of the ophthalmic division of the trigeminal nerve. In the majority of the cases, it passes through a supraorbital notch, which can be occasionally completed by a fibrous band. It can also exit through a foramen situated 1.5 mm above the supraorbital rim. Multiple exit points can be found in some patients, respectively, in 16 and 18% on the right side and left side. At this point, the nerve divides into a superficial and a deep branch, although it can split before exiting the supraorbital rim in a minority of the cases [5]. Here the nerve displays an intimate relationship with the corrugator supercilii muscle.

The traditional nerve topography was recently reviewed, and four types of branching patterns were described [5]. In 40% of the cases, the deep division only leaves strands deep to the frontalis muscle (Type I); in 34%, both divisions send branches (Type II); and in 4%, it is the superficial division that arborizes (Type III). In the rest of the cases (Type IV), the branches emerge mostly from the superficial division cranially to the corrugator muscle.

The reason why some patients do not respond to the surgical decompression of the only supraorbital nerve and need a more medial muscular resection is that the supratrochlear nerve may be involved.

The supratrochlear nerve is the smallest terminal branch of the frontal nerve, which itself originates from the ophthalmic division of the trigeminal nerve. It emerges between the trochlea and the supraorbital foramen. The exit point of the supraorbital nerve can be either a foramen or a notch, with findings of a notch present on both sides being more frequent. However it should be noted that it is also possible to discover a notch on one side and a foramina on the other or rarely a bilateral foramina; the first potential compression point of the nerve can be located here. The floor of the notch is in fact a fibrous band which surrounds the nerve. Compression symptoms appear frequently in two instances: firstly, when the nerve passes through the band itself and, secondly, when the band appears to be very thick [5].

The emergence patterns were classified in two main types. In 69% of the cases, the nerve emerges from the medial portion of the supraorbital rim independently either as a single branch (Type Ia) or as two separated branches (Type Ib). In the remaining cases, the supraorbital and the supratrochlear nerves appear to come out at the same point (Type II). Moreover, Type II was further divided into two subtypes: IIa and IIb, depending on whether the nerve emerges as a single trunk or as two branches.

The nerve then ascends through the forehead and passes through the fat pad behind the orbicularis oculi, and it pierces the corrugator muscle. The point where it enters the muscles has a mean distance of 16.4 mm from the midsagittal line and of 2.3 mm from the supraorbital rim. Furthermore, both its entrance and its exit from the muscle are possible compression points [4]. There is a significant individual variability in the relationship between the muscle and the nerve. Normally, the nerve divides into two branches within the thin retro-orbicularis oculi fatty tissue, and these branches follow four possible paths. Most commonly (84%), both branches pierce the muscle (Type I). In Type II, one branch enters the muscle, and one remains deep to the muscular plane. Type III is where both branches run deep and do not pierce the muscle. Type IV is when they leave immediately fine branches that cannot be identified [5].

Another source of compression can be the interaction of nerves with the vascular structures.

The main vessels that may be involved are the supratrochlear and the supraorbital arteries. The supratrochlear artery passes through the frontal notch and runs medial to the nerve and can be found around the medial canthal vertical line. In a third of the cases, the artery crosses underneath the nerve deep to the corrugator from medial to lateral. It then pierces the corrugator supercilii and reaches the subcutaneous layer from 15 to 25 mm above the supraorbital rim.

The supraorbital artery can be found in a vertical line corresponding to the medial limbus of the cornea, sharing its course with the supraorbital nerve.

Another vascular structure that could be involved is the frontal branch of the superficial temporary artery, which enters the frontal region at different transverse levels at the lateral orbital rim vertical line. It runs superficial to the frontalis muscle and becomes progressively more superficial moving medially [11].

2.2. Temporal region

The temporal region corresponds to the lateral part of the skull; it is a paired anatomical region lying above the zygomatic arch in front of the external ear. It is limited superiorly by the superior and inferior temporal lines and inferiorly and laterally by the zygomatic arch.

The tissues are arranged in two main layers: the superficial and the deep fascia. The superficial temporal fascia consists of a continuous layer including the galea aponeurotica, the superficial muscular aponeurotic system (SMAS) in the zygomatic and cheek region, and the platysma. It is composed by thin skin, loose areolar subcutaneous tissue, and the flat muscles. Deep to this plane, it can be found a potential space characterized by loose tissue.

http://dx.doi.org/10.5772/64652

Connecting the superficial to the deep fascia and the periosteum, there is a system of ligamentous attachments. These structures are the temporal ligamentous adhesion and the ligamentous structures that origin from it, particularly the superior temporal septum and the inferior temporal septum. They retain the superficial tissues, limiting the possibility of dissection in this area.

The superior temporal septum extends from the junction between the superficial temporal fascia and the galea toward the periosteum along the superior temporal line of the cranium. It ends 30 mm from the orbital rim providing a firm adhesion, while posteriorly it forms a septum.

The inferior temporal septum extends from the lateral corner of the temporal ligament to the external acoustic meatus, following an oblique path.

The temporal region can be divided in the upper temporal compartment, enclosed between these two septa, and the lower temporal compartment, located under the inferior temporal septum, limited inferiorly by the zygomatic arch and anteriorly by the frontal process of the zygoma.

The upper compartment is not crossed by any relevant structures, and tissues here are easy to dissect. On the contrary, the lower one presents different fibrous attachments of crisscrossed fibers. The surgical separation of these planes is harder to achieve because of these adhesions and also for the presence of multiple nervous and vascular structures, in particular branches of the superficial temporal artery.

The conflicts that may occur between the nerves and the myofascial and vascular structures could be involved in the etiopathology of temporal headache. The nerves involved are the zygomaticotemporal branch and, less frequently, the auriculotemporal branch of the trigeminal nerve. Owing to this, neurectomy and decompression of the nerves are both considered appropriate treatment for temple migraine.

Moreover, the lower temporal compartment contains the temporal branches of the facial nerve, running through the roof of the compartment parallel to the line of attachment of the inferior septum within a thin fat pad. They are predominantly located cephalad to the sometime duplicated sentinel vein, but thin inconstant nerve branches can run also caudal to it. The gross path corresponds to a line going from 0.5 cm below the tragus to a point approximately 1.5 cm above the later part of the ipsilateral eyebrow. The individual variability is very consistent, and therefore the surgical approach should be judicious, in order to spare both nervous and vascular structures [5, 6].

The zygomaticotemporal branch of the maxillary division originates from the bifurcation of the zygomatic branch of the trigeminal nerve; after crossing a canal in the zygomatic bone, it reaches the anterior part of the temporal fossa 17 mm posterolateral and 6.5 mm cephalad from the palpebral fissure; it perforates the deep temporal fascia and arborizes within the subcutaneous tissues to innervate the skin of the temporal area. There are also accessory nerves, which can be located superiorly, immediately adjacent or posterolateral to the main branch. The last one runs horizontally and connects with the auriculotemporal branch of the mandibular division.

A recent study found three potential courses for the path of the nerve from the orbit to the subcutaneous tissues. In almost 50% of the specimens, there was no intramuscular course to be found: the nerve bores the fascia within the temporal fossa. This may relate to the percentage of nonresponders to the surgical decompression. In the other cases, an intramuscular path to the temporal muscle was found for the nerve, either very short (22%) or long and tortuous (28%). In about one-third of the population, there are two branches, which in some cases (6%) pass through two different foramina [5].

Furthermore, the auriculotemporal nerve represents a minor trigger site for temple headache. It is a branch of the mandibular division of the trigeminal nerve which runs behind the temporomandibular joint adherent to the parotid gland. It then turns superiorly behind the joint and ascends over the posterior portion of the zygomatic arch. Here, it can leave up to four branches running cranially within the layers of the temporoparietal fascia.

A significant relationship with the superficial temporal artery was found in 34% of the cases: the nerve runs close to it in the soft tissues of the temple region, representing the potential vascular compression point. The artery can bifurcate below or above the superior margin of the zygomatic arch with three possible patterns. In 60% of the cases, the artery crosses the auriculotemporal nerve in one site, located approximately 107.88 mm lateral to the midline and 37.53 mm cranial to the nasion-lateral orbit line. In the other cases, either the nerve crosses the artery or they coil together for a mean length of 21 mm. This spiral interaction begins about 123 mm lateral to the midline and 25 mm cranial to the nasion-lateral orbit line and ends 117 mm lateral to the midline and 38 mm cranial to the nasion-lateral orbit line.

There are also two other trigger points associated to myofascial structures, particularly to the preauricular fascial bands in the sub-superficial fascial layer. The first one is located average of 13.1 mm anterior and 5.0 mm superior to the most anterosuperior point of the external auditory meatus, while the second is centered at an average of 11.9 mm anterior and 17.2 mm superior to the same landmark [5, 11].

2.3. Occipital region

The occipital region is an unpaired and median anatomic region corresponding to the posterior part of the cranium. It is composed of five layers: first the skin, very thick and adherent to the underlying planes; followed by a richly vascularized subcutaneous tissue, the muscular aponeurotic layer, composed of the posterior muscular bellies of the occipitalis muscle; the epicranial aponeurosis (galea aponeurotica); and then a loose areolar tissue, poor of connective tissue attachments; its laxity allows the scalp to slide on the skull and justifies the ease of surgical dissection in this area. Moreover, it is possible to create flaps without risk of damaging vessels and nerves, since these structures run in the superficial fascia [3, 5, 6].

The common occipital headache symptoms here can be caused by the compression of the greater, lesser, and third occipital nerves. This is due to the presence of muscular and fascial entrapments and also because of their interaction with the vascular structures [3, 5, 6, 12–15].

The greater occipital nerve originates from the medial branch of the C2 dorsal root. It curves to reach the occipital region, running caudal to the inferior oblique muscle and sometimes piercing it. Then it reaches the semispinalis muscle, where it is possible to identify the deepest potential compression point of the nerve. The average location is 20.13 mm from the midline and 77.38 mm inferior from the occipital protuberance [6]. The course of the nerve in the area of the superior nuchal line is variously described, because of the large anatomical variability that these structures present. According to some authors, the nerve arches medially to the semispinalis muscle, boring the fascial plane, while others describe it piercing the muscles themselves: the semispinalis in the vast majority of cases (90% of cases), the inferior oblique, or the trapezius [3, 5–11]. The latest studies have shown the exact location of the intramuscular course of the nerve: it is located 3 cm below and 1.5 cm lateral to the occipital protuberance [3, 5]. The point of muscle penetration has a mean horizontal distance from the midline of 11 mm on the left and of 11.8 mm on the right. The mean vertical distance from the line passing at the level of the lowest portion of the external auditory canals is 26 mm on the left and 27 mm on the right. The second trigger point can be found at its entrance into the deep fascia underlying the semispinalis or the muscle itself [3, 5, 6]. The third and the fourth points are located, respectively, by the entrance of the nerve in the semispinalis capitis and trapezius muscles. The fifth point of possible compression is where the nerve pierces the tendinous insertion of the trapezius into the nuchal line. In fact in the surgical decompression of the nerve, the semispinalis capitis and the trapezius together with the splenius and the occipital muscles are resected with multiple myotomies. The sixth possible compression point is related to the close relationship found between the great occipital nerve and the occipital artery in the region of the superior nuchal line. This artery is the main vessel running through the occipital area. It arises from the external carotid artery, and it runs medially to the mastoid process on the temporal bone. It then reaches the occipital region, boring the deep cervical fascia between the sternocleidomastoid and the cranial attachment of the trapezius. At this point it can be found in the subcutaneous layer leaving many convoluted branches and anastomosing with the contralateral artery [3]. In more than 50% of the cases, an intimate anatomical relationship was found. There are two possible types of interaction: they can coil together (70%) with a mean length of interaction being 37.6 mm and its caudal-most aspect a 25.34 mm from the midline and 24.91 mm caudal to the horizontal line through the occipital protuberance; the mean location of the cranial-most aspect of the artery-nerve relationship in this group was 42.09 mm from the midline and 0.97 mm caudal to the horizontal line through the occipital protuberance. The other possibility is a simple crossing (30%) with the nerve passing superficial to the artery 30.27 mm lateral to the midline and 10.67 mm caudal to the horizontal line through the occipital protuberance [3, 5, 6].

Furthermore, minor trigger sites are also described in this area [3, 5, 6]. They are related to the lesser and to the third occipital nerves, which can be similarly compressed by fascial bands and the occipital artery branches. If the lesser occipital nerve is affected, it can be responsible of laterally located pain symptoms. It arises from C2 or rarely from C3 dorsal root; it emerges from the posterior border of the sternocleidomastoids, seldom piercing it, and then ascends along it. The emergence point was found with a 3-cm diameter located 6.5 cm from midline and 5.3 cm below the line drawn between the two external auditory canals. When symptoms concern the midportion of the occipital region, the third occipital nerve is involved. It is the medial branch of the posterior division of the third cervical nerve, and it travels deeply along the semispinalis. It then exits the overlying trapezius muscle or the fasci, emerging in an area 4 cm in diameter centered 1.3 cm from midline and 6.2 cm below the line between the two external auditory canals [3, 5, 6, 11].

3. Surgical treatment of migraine

3.1. Frontal trigger site

Initially, patients who suffered from frontal migraine headache due to muscle compression underwent a procedure developed by Guyuron et al., in which hyperexcitability and inflammation of supraorbital and supratrochlear nerves were eliminated through selective myotomies of depressor supercilii, corrugator supercilii, and procerus muscles, using a transpalpebral approach. The frontal trigger site was approached by means of incising the supratarsal crease involving up to two-thirds of the medial limit of the caudal portion of the conventional upper blepharoplasty incision. After, a skin-orbicularis oculi muscle flap was raised above the level of the septum and the orbicularis muscle in a cephalic direction. The depressor supercilii muscle was exposed and resected as completely as possible, protecting the supraorbital nerve and supratrochlear nerve to allow exposure of the corrugator supercilii muscle. After excision with electrocautery of the corrugator supercilii, lateral fibers of the procerus muscle encasing the supratrochlear nerve were also removed. Fat was then harvested either from the medial fat pad of the upper lid or from an area deep to the deep temporal fascia above the zygomatic arch, if endoscopic ablation of the zygomaticotemporal branch of the trigeminal nerve was performed concomitantly, and placed to fill the depression left following

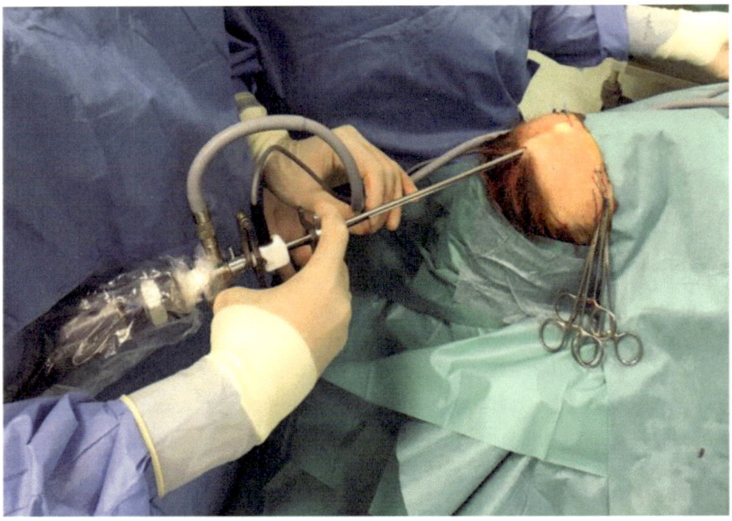

Figure 1. The endoscope is inserted through one incision in the subgaleal plane until the superciliary region is reached to perform the section of the corrugator supercilii, depressor supercilii, and procerus muscles (this picture belongs to Prof. Edoardo Raposio).

resection of the corrugator supercilii muscle and to cushion the nerves [6–8]. The supraorbital nerve, a sensory branch of the ophthalmic division of the trigeminal nerve, exits the orbit by passing over the supraorbital ridge or via a notch or foramen before diving into a superficial and deep branch and is intimately related to the corrugator supercilii in 78% of patients. While incomplete resection of the glabellar muscle group may account for persistent migraine in some patients, the supraorbital foramen (present in 25% of patients) may represent an additional compression site. Since 2002 Guyuron has performed a supraorbital foraminotomy during release of the supraorbital nerve if encountered during resection of the corrugator. As regards the effectiveness of transpalpebral nerve decompression in contrast with the endoscopic approach, a transpalpebral approach did not allow myotomies to be complete, failing to remove more than one-third of the corrugator supercilii muscle transverse portion. The whole corrugator supercilii muscle might be removed by means of an endoscopic approach, which was thus claimed to be more thorough and appropriate for this purpose. Endoscopic nerve decompression, however, was not performed on patients with long foreheads (8 cm measured from the anterior hairline to the supraorbital ridge) or on patients with significant curvature to the forehead, as endoscopic access would have been difficult to impossible. It relies on three to six access incisions 1.5–2 cm in length, located 1–2 cm behind the anterior hairline. Two distinct surgical instruments, an endoscope and a dissector, are generally used. In an effort to reduce the invasiveness of the current endoscopic techniques, we described our minimally invasive, endoscopic selective myotomy technique with a single access, performed with a specifically modified endoscope (Karl Storz, Tuttlingen, Germany) and without the need for general anesthesia [12–15]. With the patient supine and the head in a neutral position, frontal trigger nerves are located. Skin markings are drawn above the eyebrow bilaterally, at the mid-pupillary line (supraorbital nerve) and 1 cm medially (supratrochlear nerve). In this minimally invasive technique for forehead headache treatment, local anesthesia with diluted 40-cc Carbocaine 1% + 40-cc NaCl 0.9% and 20-cc sodium bicarbonate 8.4% is injected in the forehead, between the glabellar region and about 2 cm behind the anterior hairline. The infiltration of local anesthetic allows not only anesthesia but also the undermining of the tissues and the creation of a space between the periosteum and adjacent tissues to facilitate endoscopic visualization. A single 1.5-cm incision is then performed on the midline, 1 cm behind the frontal hairline. All tissues are dissected (cutaneous, subcutaneous, aponeurotic galea) until the periosteum is reached in the subgaleal plane. This location is chosen so that the postoperative scar will be hidden in the patient's hair. Tissues all over the forehead bilaterally are undermined in the subgaleal plane through the hairline incision by means of long scissors. Undermining must be done carefully, particularly when the inferior limit of the undermining area (superciliary region) is reached, in order not to damage supratrochlear and supraorbital nerves. The lateral anatomic limit of the undermining area is the temporal region, bilaterally. In order to lift the frontal skin during the endoscopic procedure and better visualize the anatomic structures, nylon 1-0 sutures are placed in the superciliary region at each side of both supratrochlear and supraorbital nerves bilaterally. Then a suction of blood and residual anesthetic fluid in the entire undermined forehead is performed through the hairline incision before inserting the endoscope and whenever the endoscopic view is not clear. Our modified endoscope (Karl Storz, Tuttlingen, Germany) consists of a 9-mm trocar with an air/insufflator/

suction triple valve, a straight Hopkins telescope with fiber-light transmission, a Wittmöser operating sheath with a connection for high-frequency diathermy, and a specifically designed elliptical-tipped wire loop electrode for electrocautery. The modified endoscope is inserted through the incision in the subgaleal plane (**Figure 1**) and used to perform endoscopically assisted section of the corrugator supercilii, depressor supercilii, and procerus muscles bilaterally (**Figure 2**), with the purpose of decompressing the supraorbital nerve and supra-trochlear nerves bilaterally. During this procedure, it is important to dissect every part of the muscle, which receives facial nerve fibers responsible for contraction of the muscle itself, in order to prevent irritation to surrounding nerves from the muscle's movement. At the end of the procedure, after an accurate hemostasis, the cutaneous access is closed with absorbable suture, without any drainage, and a compressive bandage is positioned all around the patient's head.

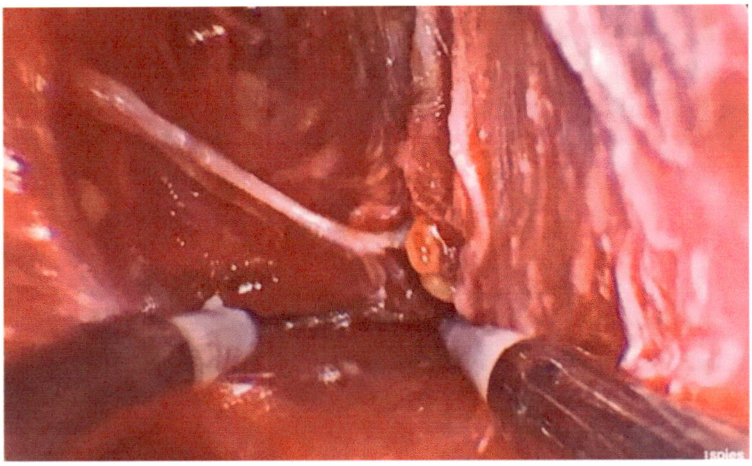

Figure 2. Endoscopically assisted section of the corrugator supercilii and depressor supercilii muscles (this picture belongs to Prof. Edoardo Raposio).

3.2. Temporal trigger site

The zygomaticotemporal branch of the trigeminal nerve travels between the temporalis muscle and the lateral orbital wall and is commonly transected during craniofacial or esthetic forehead surgery, with no reported consequence. Transcutaneous tattooing of the nerve site by the measurement from the lateral canthus (17 mm lateral and 6.5 mm cephalad to the lateral canthus) could be used to forewarn the surgeon about the location of the nerve. Under local anesthesia two incisions measuring 1.5 cm are made on each side located approximately 7 and 10 cm from the midline. Dissection under the incisions is realized by scissors to expose the deep temporal fascia and with a periosteal elevator is conducted medially, laterally, cephalad, and caudally to accommodate the endoscope. To reach this nerve safely, it is crucial to identify the deep temporal fascia beneath the scalp incision and to continue the dissection in this plane. The zygomaticotemporal branch of the trigeminal nerve is then exposed, isolated, and avulsed on one side, removing approximately 2.5 cm of the nerve, while on the other side, it is decompressed by widening the fascia opening and removing the zygomaticotemporal artery. The proximal nerve end is allowed to retract into temporalis muscle to reduce the risk of neuroma formation. Some surgeons prefer to locate the zygomaticotemporal branch of the trigeminal nerve through a transpalpebral incision [5, 6]. A careful dissection along the inferior lateral orbital rim over the deep temporal fascia is performed. The superficial temporal fascia is carefully lifted off the deep temporal fascia with an elevator and a lighted retractor to retract the tissue and protect the sentinel vein and the temporal branch of the facial nerve. Careful dissection around the vein to identify the zygomaticotemporal nerve is performed, and once identified, the zygomaticotemporal nerve is avulsed. Both avulsion neurectomy and decompression of the zygomaticotemporal branch of the trigeminal nerve are equally effective methods for the treatment of temporal migraine headache, but decompression is the first option. The avulsion remains a logical alternative when decompression is technically difficult or when the zygomaticotemporal branch of the trigeminal nerve has multiple branches without concomitant vessels or tight fascia bands. Our experience about surgical treatment of temporal migraine concerns on open decompression of the zygomaticotemporal branch of trigeminal nerve. In the first moment, the patient indicates the trigger point in temporal region, after we inject local anesthetic and we make a 3-cm cutaneous incision in the same area. By the blunt tip scissors, we perform the dissection up to the deep temporal fascia. We open the inferior temporal septum keeping above the fascia to expose the inferior temporal compartment that contains the zygomaticotemporal nerve, sentinel vessels, and temporal branches of facial nerve. After operating this septum, it is imperative that the level of dissection hug the floor of the space, that is, directly on the deep temporal fascia, because the temporal branches of facial nerve course through the roof of the lower temporal compartment immediately abutting the inferior temporal septum. Then we perform the zygomaticotemporal nerve decompression realizing it from constricting temporal muscle fibers, without any avulsion. When the patient describes a pulsing pain in the temporal region, we perform the electrocautery of sentinel vessels. Eventually, the cutaneous access is closed with absorbable suture, and a compressive bandage is positioned all around the patient's head.

3.3. Occipital trigger site

The purpose of the surgical treatment of Site IV is to remove the potential compression points of the greater occipital nerve along its course throughout the semispinalis and the trapezius muscles to the subcutaneous tissue of the occipital scalp. The avulsion of the third occipital nerve (TON) during the occipital migraine surgery does not improve clinical outcomes. When this nerve is encountered during the dissection of the GON, it is sacrificed, but the superficial compression of the TON does not contribute significantly to the onset of occipital migraine headaches. Guyuron et al. described their surgical procedure to treat occipital migraine [6]. With the patient prone, under general anesthesia, a horizontal 5- to 6-cm incision is made approximately 3 cm below the occipital protuberance. After reaching the trapezius muscle in the deep anatomical planes, a vertical incision is made over his fascia, where 1–3 mm of vertically oriented muscle fibers is present. If the avulsion of TON is performed, the third occipital nerve is allowed to retract into the portion of the semispinalis capitis muscle to avoid the scar entrapped it, causing a painful neuroma. If the trapezius muscle extends to the midline raphe, it is divided and retracted laterally, and the semispinalis muscle is then further exposed. The trunk of the GON is located usually approximately 1.5 cm from the midline and 3 cm caudal to the occipital protuberance and is identified when the dissection continues under the trapezius fascia and muscle laterally. The GON is released from surrounding muscle and any fascial bands overlying the nerve until the subcutaneous plane is reached. Furthermore, a 2-cm-long segment of the semispinalis capitis muscle between the nerve and the midline raphe is removed. When the occipital artery is ectasic and entangled with the nerve (**Figures 3–4**), the ligation is performed, and the GON is separated from the remaining muscle by placing a laterally elevated subcutaneous flap deeply to the nerve. This procedure is then repeated on the opposite side if indicated. Sometimes the muscle fibers of semispinalis capitis are splitting the nerve within; in this case they are also released. When the nerve is within the trapezial tunnel, the dissection is carried distally releasing the GON. This tunnel is the site where the greater occipital nerve penetrates through the trapezial fascial attachments to the occiput, and it has 1- to 2-cm oblique superolateral direction where it often contains angiolymphatics, another possible compression variable that is removed. Our surgical GON bilaterally decompression technique is performed under local anesthesia with the patient prone. After injecting of diluted 40-cc Carbocaine 1% + 40-cc NaCl 0.9% and 20-cc sodium bicarbonate 8.4%, a horizontal occipital scalp incision 6 cm in length is made along the superior nuchal midline to expose subcutaneous structures. No trichotomy is needed, and the scar from the incision will be hidden in the patient's hair. First of all the dissection of occipital muscle is performed; then a minute separation of the trapezius fibers expose the GON and the semispinalis capitis muscle. Trapezius and semispinalis capitis muscle are carefully undermined following the nerve course as far as possible.

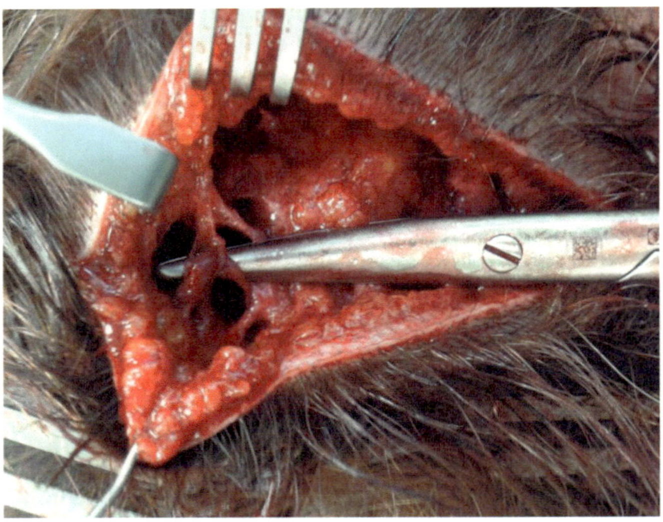

Figure 3. The dilated left occipital artery constricting the left great occipital nerve (this picture belongs to Prof. Edoardo Raposio).

http://dx.doi.org/10.5772/64652

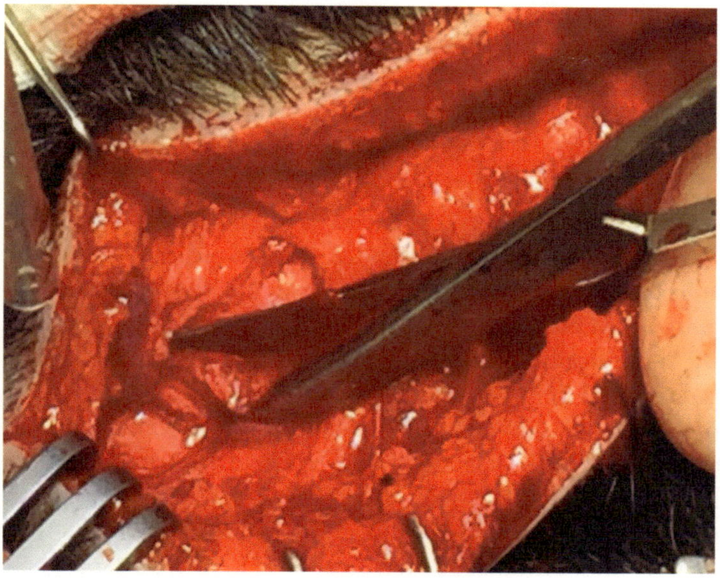

Figure 4. Aberrant left occipital arteries compressing the left occipital nerve (this picture belongs to Prof. Edoardo Raposio).

Subsequently the splenius capitis muscle, which is located laterally behind the GON, and the occipital vascular bundle are isolated from the nerve. The proximity of the occipital artery to the greater occipital nerve often seems to cause nerve compression and paroxysmal, throbbing pain. In fact, sometimes the nerve irritation that might be due to the pulsing activity of the occipital artery may be more distended than expected. In this case, the ligation of the occipital artery is performed. At the end of the procedure, after an accurate hemostasis, the cutaneous access is closed with absorbable suture, without any drainage. Presurgical planning should always include questioning for potential pain at lesser occipital nerve compression points. Furthermore, residual migraine pain after occipital nerve decompression of the greater occipital nerve may be attributable to lesser occipital nerve (LON) entrapment and should be evaluated in no responders and partial responders. The occipital artery and fascial bands along its course could potentially compress the lesser occipital nerve. If patients, in addition to compression of the GON, refer pain and symptoms specific to the lesser occipital nerve, a separate incision is made over this nerve at the posterior border of the sternocleidomastoid muscle, and it was avulsed. When a unilateral lesser occipital nerve compression is present, over the path of the LON localized along the middle third of the posterior margin of the sternocleidomastoid, laterally to the first incision of the GON, a 3-cm excision is performed. The lesser occipital nerve can be decompressed or excised and its proximal stump implanted into the muscle. When both bilateral greater occipital nerve and lesser occipital nerve decompressions are performed, two separate incisions are made, one on each side, each to access the ipsilateral greater occipital nerve and the lesser occipital nerve. As regards our experience, when trigger site is identified in the LON, a 4-cm-long lateral occipital incision is performed, followed by the dissection of occipital, trapezius, and a portion of sternocleidomastoid muscles, thus freeing the nerve. If patients present both trigger points, an 8-cm-long medial incision is made and dissection of all abovementioned muscles and vessels (occipital arteries) and isolation of both nerves are performed [15].

3.4. Auriculotemporal nerve

Auriculotemporal neuralgia has been described in the neurology literature as a syndrome "characterized by attacks of paroxysmal, moderate to severe pain on the preauricular area, often spreading to the ipsilateral temple." Chim et al. in a study concerning the anatomical variations of compression points of the auriculotemporal nerve have identified three specific points that could be surgically treated [5]. The preauricular fascial band compression points (compression points 1 and 2) in the preauricular course of the auriculotemporal nerve were found centered at 13.1 and 11.9 mm anterior and 5.0 and 17.2 mm superior to the most anterosuperior point of the external auditory meatus. The other compression point (compression point 3) is represented by the crossover in the temporal scalp between the auriculotemporal and the superficial temporal artery. Guyuron et al. developed the technique for endoscopic decompression of the zygomaticotemporal branch of the trigeminal nerve, and recently, it has been recognized that the failure of Site II surgery may be because of the lack of identification and decompression of the auriculotemporal nerve. For this reason commonly the auriculotemporal nerve decompression is performed in conjunction with the zygomaticotemporal decompression [5, 6]. We report the endoscopic surgical techniques to decompression-avulsion of the auriculotemporal nerve [5, 6, 15]. The point of maximal tenderness is marked, and Doppler findings to determinate vessel location may be used to avoid injury to the surrounding nerves or difficulty to place the endoscopic access devices. Both techniques can be combined with decompression of the trigger Site II; in that case auriculotemporal nerve is addressed first. In local anesthesia, five- to seven-port incision is designed for Site II surgery, and the 1.5-cm lateral incision is made and is extended anteriorly if necessary. Dissection to identify the vessel and nerve should be performed with blunt tip scissors along the direction of the vessel. The vessel and nerve are commonly found in the superficial layers and along the superficial temporal fascia. The use of blunt tip bipolar and regular suction is enough to safely ligate the vessel and nerve after identification. Although the area of dissection is far cephalad to the temporal branch of the facial nerve, caution should be exercised. The deep temporal fascia is then identified, and placement of endoscope is performed. If one is concerned about an unusually anterior temporal artery causing compression and pain (scars beyond the hairline or proximity to the temporal branch of the facial nerve), ligation of the main trunk of the auriculotemporal nerve in the preauricular area is chosen. The area of maximal tenderness above the temporomandibular joint, which hosts the main trunk of the auriculotemporal nerve, is accessed, and the vessel and nerve are ligated in this area. A 1.5-cm incision is performed 0.5 cm in front of the tragus and above the temporomandibular joint area with the aid of Doppler. The main trunk of the auriculotemporal nerve is identified first, and the vessel is then located in the deeper plane, commonly associated with another small nerve branch. Caution should be used to avoid injury to the facial nerve, which is deep to the dissection, and to the commonly visualized vein, which is in a more superficial plane. Even with vessel ligation in this area, auriculotemporal nerve decompression and superficial temporal artery ligation in the most lateral port should be done, if possible, because of collateral flow that may still exist. If both areas are to be decompressed, lateral port access and decompression are performed first to ensure better visualization of the artery.

4. Clinical course

As stated previously, 30% of MH patients still suffer from debilitating chronic MH since they are refractory to current medical management. Moreover, not all patients may benefit from the existing therapies due to the possible adverse events and contraindications. It's our shared opinion that patients diagnosed with MH who, despite or not conservative treatment, are still symptomatic may be eligible for the surgery [9]. Being affected by mental illness and children under 16 years are the only excluding criteria.

All procedures are minimally invasive and are performed under local-assisted anesthesia as 1-day surgery with an average surgery time of less than 1 h. No drainage needs to be positioned. Patients should keep ice on the surgical area for 24 h following surgical procedure in order to lower the risk for complication of the postoperative course (e.g., hematoma, bleeding, edema). Patients must be fasting from midnight and may start feeding again since the second hour after surgery. Patients are permitted to resume ordinary activities in 1 week and heavy exercise in 3 weeks. Patients have to medicate each two days the surgical wound with Betadine and can take a shower since the day after surgery. Stitches have to be removed on the fourteenth postoperative day. The postoperative edema of the upper lid following frontal migraine surgery is almost a certainty and resolves in the following 3/5 days, while the ecchymosis will vanish by the second postoperative week. Boric water applications three times a day may help the process of reabsorption of the edema. As the edema may move in the posterior orbicular space determining the compression of the optic nerve, patients' sight must be assessed during 12 h that follow the frontal migraine surgery in order to perform a prompt surgical decompression as soon as the patient reports changes in his/her sight. However it is just an eventual complication that currently we have never observed in our clinical practice.

Patients should fill a daily headache diary and complete MH questionnaires assessing MH parameters following surgery. The same questionnaires are given preoperatively in order to assess changes in MH. Patients may be seen after initial recovery, at 1 month, and then every 3 months for 1 year.

Almost 90% of the patients can recognize more than one MH trigger site; the surgical deactivation may be performed at all sites during the same surgical procedure [10]. However, we routinely deactivate the main trigger site first, and then a second or third surgery is performed at the remaining sites 3 months after each surgery.

MH recurrence may occur from 1 up to 3 months after surgery; thus the result may be regarded as permanent only after the third postoperative month [5, 6, 9]. The frontal area has the highest rate of MH relapse [5, 6, 9].

Furthermore, patients should be informed when signing the informed consent that deactivation of a MH trigger site may unmask secondary headaches in almost 17.8% of patients and that more than one surgery may be needed [9].

5. Results

In 2000, Guyuron was the first to show in a retrospective study the relation between MH and corrugator supercilii muscle resection when he reported that 80% of patients described elimination or improvement in their headaches following corrugator supercilii muscle avulsion for forehead rejuvenation surgery [4]. This evidence was followed by a prospective study where he reported a 95% rate of either complete alleviation or improvement in MH after a mean follow-up of 1 year [5]. Over the last 15 years, Guyuron conducted several anatomical and clinical studies reporting a reduction of the frequency, duration, and intensity of MH by at least half in 80–90% of patients [4–10]. In 2011, Guyuron et al. published a study examining the long-term benefits of migraine surgery where it was reported an 88% success rate after a 5-year follow-up (29% completely healed; 59% gained improvement; 12% did not show any change) [8]. Other independent groups reported similar findings using Guyuron's protocols, demonstrating the effectiveness of the procedure and the reproducibility of the results [5, 12–15].

From June 2011 till February 2016, we have performed MH decompression surgery over 89 patients with either frontal, occipital, or temporal migraine trigger sites. After a mean follow-up of 17 months (range: 3–56 months), 93.9% of patients reported positive response to surgery, 52.4% had complete elimination of their migraine, while 41.5% referred at least a 50% reduction in MH symptoms, and 6.1% of patients did not notice any improvement after the surgery. Patients with frontal migraine trigger site reported a 94% positive response to surgery (32% complete relief and 62% significant improvement), 6% had no change in their symptoms, while patients with occipital migraine had positive response in 93.7% (85.5% complete relief and 8.2% significant improvement), and 6.3% did not get any better. Patients complaining for temporal MH had 83.3% positive surgical outcome (50% complete MH elimination, 33.3 significant improvement), and 16.7% of patients did not notice any improvement.

Overall response rates are almost the same as no significant differences can be found between the trigger sites. However, occipital migraine surgery leads to higher rates of complete relief of symptoms than the frontal and temporal and intranasal ones (85.5 vs. 32, 50, and 34%, respectively). This may be attributable to a more complete and thorough decompression since the fourth- and sixth-site surgeries are technically easier to perform.

All patients continue to experience a quality of life better than before surgery, and all would have the surgery again.

As reported in literature, we do have patients that reported complete relief during the first 30–60 days postoperatively and then gradual (though improved) return of symptoms to the treated region [5, 6, 9]. This event was most common with frontal migraine. The recurrent headaches were often described as less intense and more "treatable," and improvement were beyond baseline. These events were very disappointing for both the surgeon and the patients; no exact mechanism has been found, but it seemed to coincide directly with returning nerve function.

Average frequency, intensity, and duration of migraine headache significantly improve. The mean number of days lost from work usually reduces by four times.

Since surgical deactivation of peripheral sensory nerves has demonstrated to be effective for the treatment of MH, positive surgical outcome also has significant economic value as it leads to cost savings by cutting expenses associated with medications, doctor visits, and other financial burdens relating to migraine headache [2]. The median total cost for MH treatment drops from $5,820/year preoperatively to $900/year postoperatively with a total median cost reduction of $3,949.70/year postoperatively [2]. Surgery has a mean cost of $8,378; thus, MH surgery is cost-effective, reducing both direct and indirect cost; it has also essential social effects by improving the working performances and increasing the participation in daily living activities.

Our results are similar to those reported in literature by other authors [3, 6, 8, 9]. Global positive response rates did not show any significant differences, ranging between 80 and 95%; frontal MH is the most frequent one, but it's also the one that more often either recurred or unmasked a second trigger site after decompression surgery [8, 9]. Occipital MH instead has the better surgical outcome with the highest resolution rate [6, 8].

We believe that this difference may be caused by the compression of the dilated occipital vessels, which is often observed during the surgery and, once removed, lowers the risk for recurrence. Compression over frontal and temporal trigger site is usually consequent to muscular impingement; thus scar tissue might connect again the divided muscular fibers recreating some kind of nerve compression.

Elimination rate of frontal migraine has the highest variability, performed either by endoscopic or transpalpebral approach. Poggi reported a 16.7% complete elimination rate of frontal MH, Guyuron described a 57.1 resolution rate, while Janis gained complete relief of frontal MH only in 8.7% of patients [5]. This discrepancy may partially be explained by variation in the technique: Guyuron and Poggi performed the frontal glabellar muscle avulsion, while Janis resected the only corrugator [5, 6]. Bearden and coworkers reported 58% complete relief of frontal MH following transpalpebral corrugator muscle resection [5]. We have reported a 32% resolution of frontal MH by means of endoscopic resection of glabellar muscles. Thus, complete avulsion of procerus, corrugator, and depressor supercilii muscles may lead to higher elimination rate, but no clear evidences have been reported.

Complete resection of the glabellar muscles can be easily obtained thanks to the magnification offered by the endoscopic technique, which provides a better means to preserve the nerves, resect the muscles, and identify secondary nerve branches [12–15]. Nevertheless, patients that undergo transpalpebral access surgery may experience higher rate of complication (e.g., risk for intraoperative bleeding, more noticeable scars) and a more invasive procedure than if it would have been performed endoscopically; furthermore, patients show lower compliance to receive an open surgery. Therefore, we agree with the common belief that the endoscopic approach for frontal migraine therapy should be considered as the first choice since it has been demonstrated that odds ratio for improvement or elimination is higher if compared with the transpalpebral access [4–6, 12–15]. Trans-palpebral nerve decompression should be performed when a forehead length of 8 cm or more contraindicates the endoscopic approach.

Chepla and coworker showed that patients presenting supraorbital foramen instead of the supraorbital notch experienced higher success rate after resection of the glabellar muscle group with foraminotomy, thus supporting the hypothesis that the supraorbital nerve may be constricted within the foramen leading to frontal migraine headaches [5].

Furthermore, it emerged that some factors may affect the surgical outcome. Migraine surgery failure seems to be associated with increased intraoperative bleeding, surgery on fewer trigger sites, and history of significant head and neck trauma, while older age of migraine onset, higher rate of visual symptoms, surgery at Site I or II, and deactivating all four operative sites are associated with migraine surgery success [5, 8, 9]. The exact relationship between history of head and neck trauma, age of onset, visual symptoms, and response to surgery is not understood. Patients complaining multiple trigger sites will undergo multiple decompression surgeries addressing even minor triggers; this is likely the explanation for better outcome associated with greater number of operative locations. Intraoperative bleeding may interfere with optimal surgical outcome by promoting scar tissue formation. Intraoperative bleeding and blood pressure must be controlled aggressively in order maximize success rate. MH characteristics (e.g., frequency, duration, and amount of drugs needed) also seem to affect the surgical outcome; milder MH have higher chances of improvement in comparison to more severe ones, which are more likely to recur postoperatively [5, 8, 9]. Preliminary Botox infiltration does not affect the surgical success [10].

6. Complications

Migraine surgery is regarded as a minimally invasive procedure; thus, no concerning side effects are usually reported.

All patients undergoing frontal decompression surgery with endoscopic approach will experience frontal and upper eyelid edema of various degrees. Usually the edema resolves by the fifth postoperative day. Ecchymosis of both upper and lower eyelids and zygotic regions also follows surgery and usually vanishes by the second postoperative week. No treatment needs to be given as these collateral events resolve by themselves; boric water applications three times a day may help the process of reabsorption of the edema. As previously stated, the only hypothetical serious complication that may occur within the 12 h following the surgery is the compression of the optical nerve due to the drop of the edema into the posterior orbicular space whenever the subgaleal dissection is carried out beyond the orbital rim. Prompt recognition of patient's sight modification is mandatory in order to urgently decompress the optic nerve. Decreased glabellar muscle activity till complete elimination may occur depending on the technique applied. Slight asymmetric eyebrow movement may be also noted [6]. Patients with particularly thin skin of the frontal region may develop postoperative burn-like scar (2%) as a consequence of the endoscopic electrocautery.

Any nerve avulsion may be associated with the formation of neuromas [5]. Nevertheless, avulsion of neither the zygomaticotemporal nor the auriculotemporal branches of the trigeminal nerve is reported to lead to the formation of neuromas [5, 8].

Temporarily anesthesia occurs in all patients, which lasts 163 days on average [5, 8, 12–15]. Other minor and transient complications reported are lasting occipital numbness at 1 year (5.7%), intense itching after surgery (5.7%), hypertrophic scar (2.7%), incisional cellulitis (1%) that resolve with oral antibiotics, transient mild incisional alopecia or hair thinning (5%), lasting neck stiffness at 1 year (9%), postoperative epistaxis (4.8%), early sinusitis in the recovery period following septum and turbinate surgery (4.8), and slight septal deviation recurrence (12.9%) [3, 5, 8, 9, 12–15]. Almost 54% of patients undergoing temporal surgery reported slight hollowing of the temple [5]. All patients that were refractory to surgery did not report worsening in their MH at any follow-up. Since the operation does not cause any serious complications or side effects, it can be recommended to patients with severe forms of migraine and symptoms of drug dependency. These patients still have a 50% chance of responding with partial or even total relief of their headaches.

Author details

Edoardo Raposio*, Nicolò Bertozzi, Chiara Bordin and Francesco Simonacci

*Address all correspondence to: edoardo.raposio@unipr.it

Cutaneous, Mininvasive, Regenerative and Plastic Surgery Unit, Parma University Hospital, Plastic Surgery Chair, University of Parma, Parma, Italy

References

[1] World Health Organization. The Global Burden of Disease, 2004 Update. World Health Organization; Geneva, Switzerland; 2004.

[2] Faber C, Garcia RM, Davis J, Guyuron B. A socioeconomic analysis of surgical treatment of migraine headaches. Plast Reconstr Surg. 2012;129:871–877.

[3] Chmielewski L, Liu MT, Guyuron B. The role of occipital artery resection in the surgical treatment of occipital migraine headaches. Plast Reconstr Surg. 2013;131:351e–356e.

[4] Guyuron B, Varghai A, Michelow BJ, Thomas T, Davis J. Corrugator supercilii muscle resection and migraine headaches. Plast Reconstr Surg. 2000;106:429–437.

[5] Janis JE, Barker JC, Javadi C, Ducic I, Hagan R, Guyuron B. A review of current evidence in the surgical treatment of migraine headaches. Plast Reconstr Surg. 2014;134:131–141.

[6] Guyuron B, Kriegler JS, Davis J, Amini SB. Comprehensive surgical treatment of migraine headaches. Plast Reconstr Surg. 2005;115(1):1–9.

[7] Guyuron B, Reed D, Kriegler JS, Davis J, Pashmini N, Amini S. A placebo-controlled surgical trial of the treatment of migraine headaches. Plast Reconstr Surg. 2009;124:461–468.

[8] Guyuron B, Kriegler JS, Davis J, Amini SB. Five-year outcome of surgical treatment of migraine headaches. Plast Reconstr Surg. 2011;127:603–608.

[9] Punjabi A, Brown M, Guyuron B. Emergence of secondary trigger sites after primary migraine surgery. Plast Reconstr Surg. 2016;137:712e–716e.

[10] Guyuron B, Nahabet E, Khansa I, Reed D, Janis JE. The current means for detection of migraine headache trigger sites. Plast Reconstr Surg. 2015;136:860–867.

[11] Tolhurst DE, Carstens MH, Greco RJ, Hurwitz DJ. The surgical anatomy of the scalp. Plast Reconstr Surg. 1998;102:478.

[12] Caruana G, Bertozzi N, Boschi E, Grieco MP, Grignaffini E, Raposio E. Endoscopic forehead surgery for migraine therapy: personal technique. Ann Ital Chir. 2014;85:583–586.

[13] Raposio E, Caruana G. Frontal endoscopic myotomies for chronic headache. J Craniofac Surg. 2015;26:201–213.

[14] Caruana G, Grignaffini E, Raposio E. Endoscopic forehead muscle resection for nerve decompression: a modified procedure. Plast Reconstr Surg Glob Open. 2015;7(3):e342.

[15] Raposio E, Caruana G. Minimally invasive endoscopic surgical treatment of headache. In: Atlas of Endoscopic Plastic Surgery (Raposio E., Ed.), Springer; New York; 2016; 17–23.

Chapter 7

Surgical Management of Migraine Headaches

Michael Chung, Kyle Sanniec, Xingchen Li and
Bardia Amirlak

Additional information is available at the end of the chapter

http://dx.doi.org/10.5772/66229

Abstract

Although migraines are experienced by a significant portion of the population, current medical therapies often fail to completely alleviate the symptoms of many migraine sufferers, leading to significant residual disability. Within the last decade, migraine surgery has arisen as a viable option for patients who have exhausted all other medical treatments. Despite early resistance in the headache care community, it has become more accepted due to an increasing number of studies demonstrating efficacy and safety, and increasing evidence supporting the influence of peripheral nerves in the progression of migraine pathophysiology. Yet, it remains crucial to carefully select appropriate surgical candidates based on the assessment of various factors such as medication use, pain distribution, and any other medical conditions that may contribute to headache. It is equally important to ensure that the patient has a strong relationship with a neurologist for optimal medical management and postoperative medical support. After the appropriate trigger sites are identified, various techniques can be used to decompress the involved larger nerves, avulse the smaller nerves, and address any intranasal pathology that could be causing migraines.

Keywords: migraine surgery, chronic headache, nerve decompression, greater occipital nerve, lesser occipital nerve, occipital neuralgia, auriculotemporal nerve, zygomaticotemporal branch of the trigeminal nerve, supraorbital nerve, supratrochlear nerve

1. Introduction

Migraine headaches (MH) affect over 37 million people in the United States [1]. One in four households will have at least one person experienced migraines, as the prevalence for females reaches as high as 18%, and males 6% [2]. Sufferers can develop severe disability that takes away their ability to do even the most routine daily activities. Many do not seek treatment, and even if they do, traditional medications often fail to completely treat patients, leaving them with significant residual disability. It is estimated that one-third of migraine patients are refractory to preventative and pharmacological treatments [3]. A common and effective option for these patients is surgical decompression, which may be the only treatment that can provide permanent relief.

2. Pathophysiology

Because migraine headache development seems to be complex and multifactorial, its exact pathophysiology is complicated and incompletely understood. Classically, migraine headaches were described as a central nervous system event, but recent publications have stressed the role of peripheral nerves [4, 5]. As the evidence for a peripheral explanation of migraine development continues to increase, so does the evidence for surgical decompression as an effective treatment [6–11].

There are four commonly accepted and experimentally substantiated theories that incorporate both central and peripheral nervous system activity. These include: *periaqueductal gray matter dysfunction, interictal cortical derangement, cortical spreading depression,* and *trigeminal nerve irritation*. The combined effect of these neural derangements is a cycle of nerve irritation, inflammation, and sensory hypersensitivity in the peripheral nerve [12–14]. In migraine headaches, these derangements occur in the areas of trigeminal innervation. A recent microscopic and proteomic analysis indicated that there are indeed biostructural differences in myelin between some peripheral nerves excised from migraine patients and peripheral nerves excised from patients without migraines [15].

One theory that explains the cycle of trigeminal irritation and hypersensitization is the anatomical relationship between peripheral nerves and surrounding musculature. Trigger points for nerve irritation are located at points of intersection between nerve and muscle. One specific example is the interaction between the supratrochlear and supraorbital nerve branches of the ophthalmic division of the trigeminal nerve and the corrugator and depressor supercilii muscle [16]. The observation that many patients with frontal migraines have supercilii hypertrophy supports the theory that muscle impaction on the nerve at least plays a role in inducing migraine pain [17]. Furthermore, the beneficial effect of onabotulinumtoxinA injection into this muscle group reinforces this notion [18, 19]. Other trigger sites of nerve and muscle interaction include the zygomaticotemporal branch of the maxillary division of the trigeminal nerve as it pierces the temporal muscle and the greater occipital nerve (GON) as it passes through the splenius capitus muscle.

3. Surgical treatment

3.1. Rationale and indication for surgical treatment

In the last century, several surgeons demonstrated the effects of operating on nerves to treat migraine headaches. From these studies, they noticed some beneficial results, but the

http://dx.doi.org/10.5772/66229

morbidity and adverse sequelae were unacceptable to further this practice. The first attempt to treat MH was conducted by Walter Dandy in 1931, who removed the inferior cervical and first thoracic sympathetic ganglions [20]. In 1946, Gardner resected the greater superficial petrosal nerve in 26 patients [21]. Despite having some reduction in symptoms, he reported complications such as nasal dryness, decreased tear production, and corneal ulceration. A few decades later, temporal neurovascular bundle resection and greater occipital nerve resection were reported by Murillo [22] and Murphy [23]. While innovative, these surgeries were radical and led to numerous side effects like numbness and muscle weakness. Despite the unwanted effects from surgery, these studies showed potential and provided the groundwork for modern surgical treatment of migraine headaches.

With better understanding of migraine pathophysiology and advancements in technology and surgical techniques within the last two decades, surgical methods of treating migraine headaches have been demonstrated to indeed be significantly useful [4]. As the pioneer of modern surgical decompression for migraine headaches, Guyuron observed that among his patients who underwent cosmetic forehead rejuvenation, a number of those with preoperative migraine headaches received complete elimination or significant reduction in headache symptoms [16]. In this forehead rejuvenation surgery, the glabellar muscle group (corrugator, depressor supercilii, and procerus) is resected. As anatomical studies show that the supraorbital and supratrochlear nerves are intimately associated with this muscle group. Therefore, if nerve irritation from this relationship contributes significantly to the pathophysiology of migraine headaches, resection of the muscle group at this site theoretically should resolve symptoms [24]. This led to a retrospective report, and eventually a prospective double-blinded sham-controlled study, as a protocol for surgical migraine treatment was developed [16, 24]. A five-year retrospective follow-up study confirmed that 88% of these patients, who underwent this prospective trial, experienced a positive response to the surgery. Specifically, 29% reported complete elimination of all migraine symptoms [9]. In time, the recognition of additional extracranial trigger sites and several retrospective studies demonstrated significant efficacy in reducing migraine symptoms [6, 8–11, 16, 24, 25]. The combination of numerous studies shows that on average success from decompression surgery, meaning at least 50% reduction in symptoms, nears 90% [4]. As many as 63% of patients report complete elimination of migraine symptoms [9, 26–28]. As mentioned earlier, there are structural differences in the myelin sheath of some of the nerves excised from migraine patients versus those without migraines [15]. This biostructural difference suggests a peripheral mechanism in migraine pathology and thus further supports the rationale for surgical removal or decompression of these nerves. Finally, the sham controlled study conducted by Guyuron provides evidence against the placebo effect explanation [9, 25].

3.2. Migraine trigger site decompression surgery: arguments for and against

Following the first successful report by Guyuron in 2002, migraine trigger site deactivation surgery has been received with some controversy in neurology. Our understanding of migraine headache's complex pathophysiology and how interactions between central and peripheral mechanisms influence the development of migraine headaches is an ongoing investigation. The unclear mechanism of action in the context of current migraine pathophysiology models, and the potential for serious irreversible adverse events, causes uncertainty and hesitation among certain headache care providers. It is possible that procedures involving nerve avulsions or possible damage to nerves may result in numbness, paresthesias, dysesthesias, and exacerbated pain postoperatively [29, 30]. However, studies have shown few nonserious complications, often limited locally to the surgical site, and no complications requiring a return to the operating room [4]. Criticisms against surgical treatments also point to possible weaknesses and design flaws in early key studies that show significant efficacy from surgical deactivation [31]. Due to the nature of long-term surgical trials, it is very difficult to design studies that can both satisfy the biggest skeptics and also remain ethical in what patients are required to undergo through the course of the trial. Even so, evidence supporting the migraine decompression surgery is accumulating at a rapid pace. In addition to over 30 anatomical studies to date, there are 17 clinical studies, including a sham control prospective trial, showing the positive effect of decompression surgery and its long-term efficacy [4]. Nevertheless, migraine pathophysiology is complex and dynamic. It is unclear the role of surgical decompression in chronic migraine patients with triggers that may be predominantly central. In each study, certified neurologists were intimately involved throughout every step of each trial [32]. Therefore, it is critical that every patient being evaluated for migraine surgical decompression is also concurrently evaluated by a neurologist to ensure the best understanding of the unique mechanistic picture of their headaches. The cooperation between neurologists and plastic surgeons in each step of treatment for migraine patients is essential: from diagnosis to medication management to postoperative management.

3.3. Long-term results

A recent systematic review compiled the clinical results of all studies on migraine decompression across multiple institutions [4]. In all but one study in this review, follow-up of surgical decompression patients exceeded 1 year, with every study demonstrating sustained long-term benefits from surgery. In his review, Janis reported the average success rate of, meaning at least 50% reduction in migraine symptoms, about 90%. A five-year outcomes report on the Guyuron randomized-placebo-controlled study demonstrated both sustained benefits from surgery and a lack of serious long-term adverse complications [9]. While the placebo effect for migraine surgery is possible, it is unlikely that it is so significant 5 years after intervention. This five-year study, and the other studies reviewed by Janis, provides evidence for the sustained, long-term benefits of migraine decompression surgery, with minimal risk for serious complications [4, 9, 25, 28, 33].

3.4. Preoperative considerations

Before taking a migraine patient to undergo surgical intervention, there are several considerations that the headache care provider should use to identify the ideal candidate. It is of upmost importance for the patient to see a neurologist to confirm the diagnosis. A headache questionnaire and patient headache log can be very useful in identifying the migraine patient. Equally as important, the neurologist can help manage the numerous migraine medications that patients often take. It is important to control the use of narcotics to prevent medication overuse headache or even a reduced response to surgery. Narcotic users showed significantly less improvement in frequency, duration, and severity of migraines in a 2014 study [26]. On

Site I—Frontal headache	Site II—Temporal headache
Frontal pain Stress Robust muscles for frowning Eyebrow/eyelid ptosis Tenderness Corrugator contraction triggered by intense and bright lights (sunglasses often needed)	Temporal pain Morning peak Stress Clenching/grinding Trigger point tenderness TMJ pain
Site III—Rhinogenic headache	**Site IV—Occipital headache**
Retroorbital pain Early morning peak Change in weather related Allergy related Hormone related Rhinorrhea Cyclic	Occipital pain No specific time when pain is worst Stress Related to heavy exercise Muscle tightness Trigger point tenderness Radiation of pain to retroorbital area or area above the posterior superior part of the ear

Table 1. Constellation of symptoms for each common trigger site [36].

physical exam and history, there should be evidence of nerve irritation as evidenced by tenderness in the specific topographic compression sites. Additionally, there should be no other medical or neurological conditions that may likely explain another cause for their headache symptoms. Assess for any unacceptable surgical risk. Pregnant and nursing women are typically not considered for surgical intervention.

The headache care provider is led to suspect various trigger sites for the cause of the patient's pain by considering the constellation of symptoms. This is outlined in **Table 1**. The patient can usually give an idea of where the pain originates and where it spreads to. On palpation, tender areas often correspond with anatomically studied nerve compression sites. For intranasal sources of pain, the nose can be examined in office by a direct or indirect endoscopic approach to identify septal deviations or masses such as turbinate hypertrophy and concha bullosa. These findings can be confirmed by X-ray computed tomography. Typically, after confirmation of migraine by a neurologist, patients undergo BOTOX injections in each of the identified sites to temporarily relieve symptoms. Targeted chemodenervation by this toxin is also used to confirm the sites suspected to benefit from surgical excision [17, 34]. An alternative method is chemical nerve block. Local anesthesia is often used by surgeons to identify which sites will respond to decompression. Although chemodenervation is a useful prognostic indicator for surgical success, the constellation of symptoms based on physical exam and history is just as effective at predicting which sites will benefit [35].

4. Trigger sites

There are six major trigger sites identified by careful anatomical studies and experience with migraine surgery. **Site I** refers to the frontal area migraines, where the glabellar muscles, fascial bands, supraorbital and supratrochlear vessels, and at times supraorbital foraminal anatomy (foramen versus notch) compress the supraorbital and supratrochlear nerves (**Figure 1**). **Site II** refers to headaches originating in the temple areas of the zygomaticotemporal branch of the trigeminal nerve (ZTBTN) (**Figure 2**). The zygomaticotemporal branch of the trigeminal nerve is irritated by the temporalis muscle and accompanying fascial elements. **Site III** refers to an intranasal origin. Septal deviation with boney spurs, turbinate pathology, or bullosa anomalies causes contact with the septum. This paranasal and retrobulbar type pain is caused by irritation of terminal branches of the trigeminal nerve via the sphenopalatine, anterior ethmoidal, and posterior ethmoidal nerves (**Figure 3**). **Site IV** refers to headaches originating around the greater occipital nerve in the occipital area of the neck. In this area, the semispinalis capitis muscle, accompanying fascia, trapezius fascia, and occipital vessels can irritate and compress the greater occipital nerve. **Site V** refers to auriculotemporal nerve irritation in the temple above the temporomandibular joint (TMJ) by fascial bands, and higher in the temple by the temporal artery. **Site VI** refers to pain originating lower in the neck from the lesser occipital nerve (LON) as it is compressed by fascial and vascular elements. Each of these sites is well understood, and multiple locations of potential compression have been elucidated. In addition to the six common sites, neurologists and plastic surgeons often

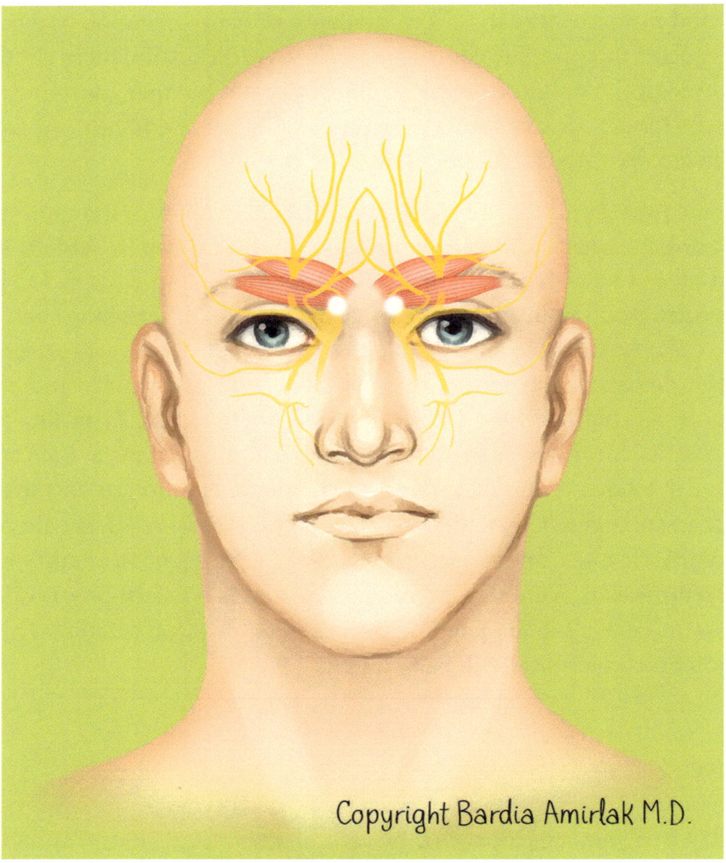

Figure 1. Site I trigger site. The supraorbital and supratrochlear nerves are found here along with the glabellar muscles, fascial bands, supraorbital and supratrochlear vessels, and possible supraorbital foramen.

http://dx.doi.org/10.5772/66229

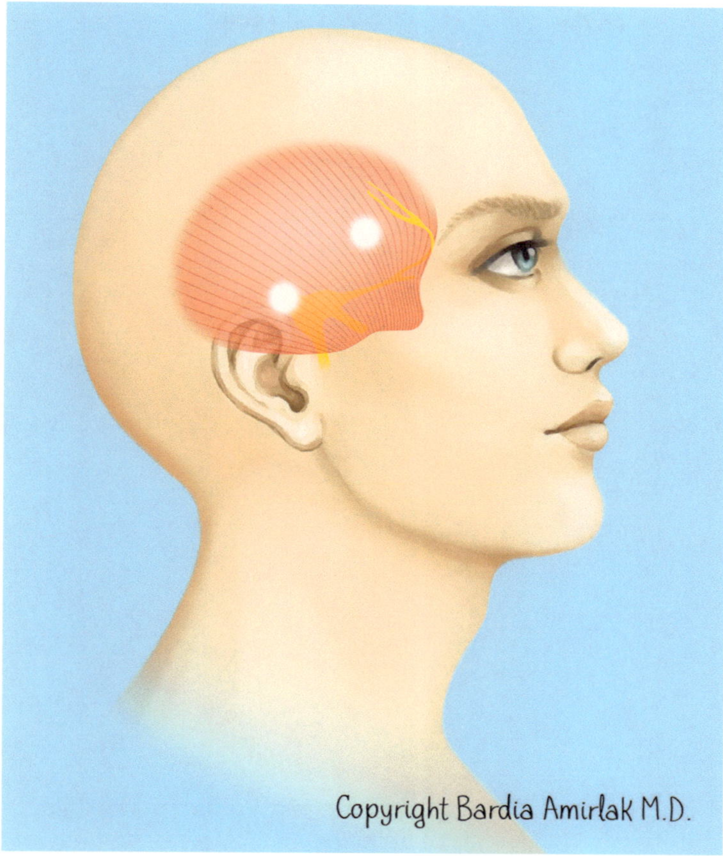

Figure 2. Site II trigger site. The zygomaticotemporal branch of the trigeminal nerve travels through the temporal muscle before piercing the deep temporal fascia 17 mm lateral and 0.6 mm superior to the lateral canthus.

encounter migraines originating from other less common sites, such as the third occipital nerve and distal tail ends of the greater and lesser occipital nerves.

4.1. Frontal triggers

Site I decompression can be approached endoscopically through multiple hairline incisions or directly through transpalpebral incision. Decompression at this site involves release of the corrugator myofascial unit by partial resection of the corrugator supercilii muscle (CSM) group. Alternatively, the entire glabellar muscle group can be excised, including the corrugator supercilii, depressor supercilii, and procerus muscles. Compressing fascial bands are lysed. Foraminotomy and vascular lysis are performed if necessary.

4.1.1. Transpalpebral approach

After initiation of anesthesia, the upper tarsal crease is marked on each eyelid. An incision of 1-inch length is made and extended through the orbicularis muscle. As the dissection plane is extended, several muscles come into view. Careful exposure of the depressor supercilii and

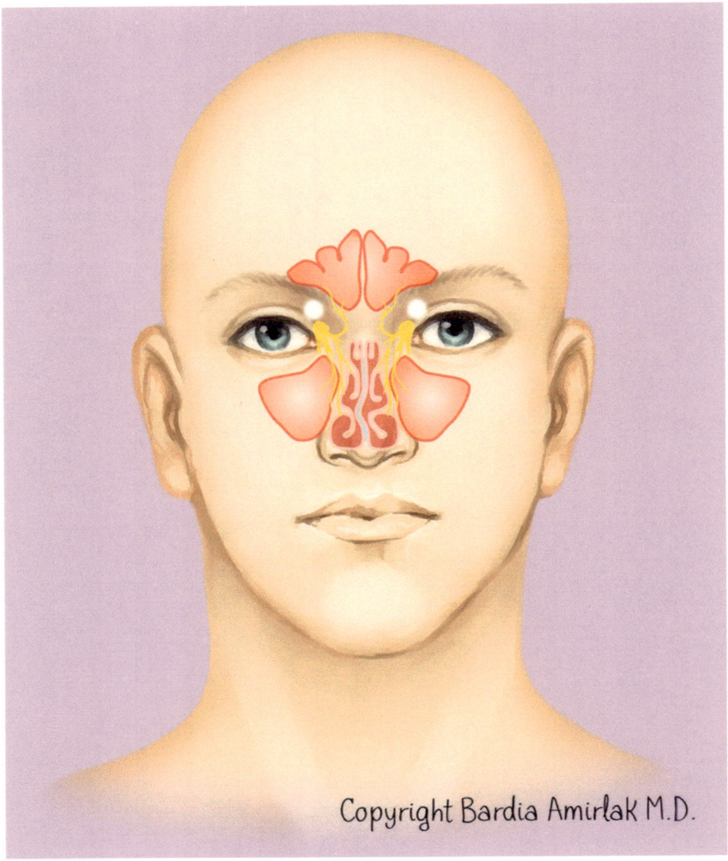

Figure 3. Site III trigger site, intranasal trigger site. The sphenopalatine, anterior ethmoidal, and/or posterior ethmoidal nerves can become irritated by structures such as a deviated septum with contact points, boney spurs with contact points to hypertrophied turbinates, or concha bullosa that lead to paranasal and retrobulbar pain.

corrugator supercilii muscles allow for thorough removal. The supraorbital nerve is encountered laterally and the supratrochlear nerve more medially. A branch of the supratrochlear artery is removed, as well as the procerus muscle. To fill the empty space, autologous fat is grafted and sutured in place.

Complications from this procedure include forehead and frontoparietal paresthesia. Although this is common, it will almost always resolve in time if the nerves are preserved in place. Even in cases of traction avulsion of the Supratrochlear nerve (STN), with the Supraorbital nerve (SON) preserved, incidents of painful neuroma are extremely rare.

4.1.2. Endoscopic approach

Five total incisions are made: one midline and two on either side of the temple. This approach allows for multiple procedures to be combined: frontal decompression and temporal ZTBTN avulsion. Therefore, this endoscopic approach is often preferred and in fact has a higher success rate, which is likely due to increased visualization and the ability to address accessory nerves. Similar to the transpalpebral approach, dissection is extended to expose the SON, STN, and surrounding musculature. The corrugator should be adequately removed and fat grafted into the area.

Complications of this approach include alopecia at port sites, which is very rare. Paresthesia of the temporal and scalp region can occur, but most resolve over time. In this area, the temporal branch of the facial nerve can theoretically be injured, resulting in paralysis of the frontalis. However, there have been no reports of this potential complication among the endoscopic surgeons. Therefore, it is important that only a well-trained and seasoned endoscopic plastic surgeon attempt this operation.

4.2. Temporal triggers

Decompression at the temporal site can be part of the endoscopic approach. The dissection is extended in the plane of the periosteum and carried to the lateral part of the supraorbital rim, lateral orbital rim, and over the deep layer of temporal fascia to the zygomatic arch, and malar arch. The ZTBTN emerges from the temporalis muscle approximately 17 mm lateral and 6 mm superior to the lateral canthus. It is found superficial to the deep temporal fascia [37]. The ZTBTN can be avulsed or decompressed, each with similar rates of surgical success [33]. As mentioned, there are no reports of neuroma with traction avulsion.

Rarely, complications from this procedure include temporary paresthesia and anesthesia. Alopecia can occur at port sites and sites of local anesthetic injection. Facial nerve injury, as mentioned above, is a theoretical complication.

The auriculotemporal nerve (AT) is addressed by decompression with a small 1 cm incision in the high temple over the compression site of the temporal artery, with or without traction avulsion of the nerve in the periauricular area and ligation of the temporal artery (Amirlak's approach) [38]. Similarly, low rates of temporary paresthesia and minor anesthesia have been reported, without reports of facial nerve injury. However, this incision in the periauricular area possesses a higher likelihood of inadvertent injury to the temporal branch of the facial nerve. Therefore, a nerve stimulator is used during surgery confirm the identities of encountered nerves.

4.3. Occipital triggers

In the preoperative waiting room, markings are made at the midline, at the hairline, and at points of maximum tenderness. After initiation of anesthesia, the patient's hair is shaved to expose the surgical area. A midline incision is made. At this point, efforts should be made to keep the incision within hair-bearing areas to prevent visible scarring. As the dissection is extended, fibers of the trapezius and semispinalis capitus muscles are differentiated. In most cases, the third occipital nerve is encountered during dissection. Although this nerve is usually avulsed when encountered, evidence has shown that there is no difference in surgical success whether or not the nerve is taken [39]. The semispinalis is further exposed by retraction. The trunk of the greater occipital nerve (GON) is located roughly 3 cm below the occipital protuberance and 1.5 cm lateral from the midline. After the nerve and surrounding musculature are identified and exposed, a full thickness section of the semispinalis is resected medial to the path of the GON. This excision is complete when the nerve is completely released, and no muscle tissue remains medial to the nerve. Superiorly, a portion of the trapezius fascia and muscle are removed, along with any fascial bands encountered on the nerve. The trapezium tunnel is opened and decompressed. An endoscopic modification of the Guyuron technique was described by the senior author (BA), which further elucidates the dynamic compression of the occipital vessels on the nerve (manuscript in preparation). Most of these vessels are lysed with no complications. Finally, a subcutaneous fat flap is passed underneath the nerve and sutured in place to protect the nerve from further compression. **Figure 4** shows the greater occipital nerve after partial decompression (opening of the trapezius fascia proximally and removal of the medial portion of the semispinalis muscle to expose the body of the nerve show that the right GON is more flat and compressed than the left).

The lesser occipital nerve (LON) is addressed similarly, but it possesses a more complicated and ill-defined anatomy. However, several approaches, including traction neurectomy, the decompression and crush technique, and the cut and burying in the muscle technique, have been described with no clear benefit of one over the other.

Temporary paresthesia and anesthesia have been reported, which improve over time.

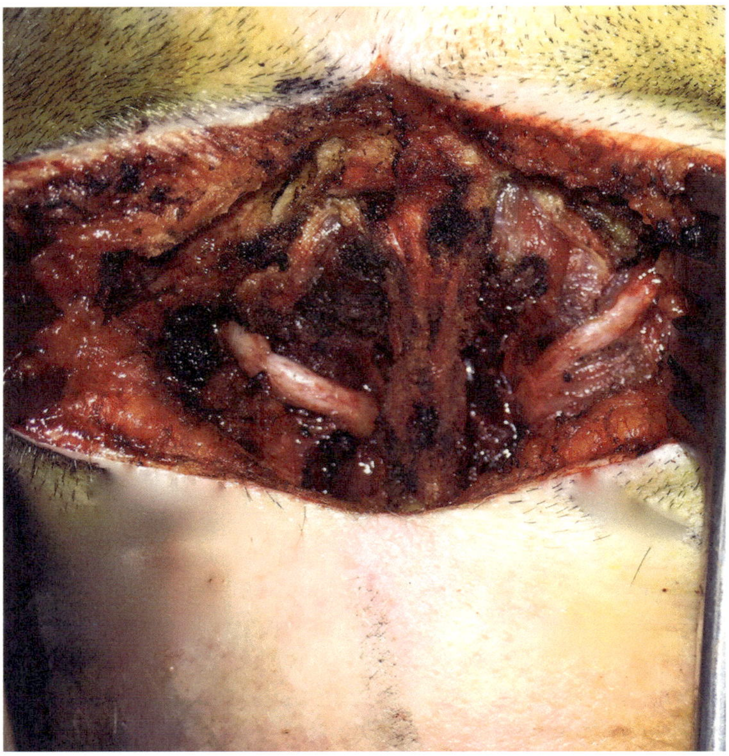

Figure 4. Intraoperative view of the greater occipital nerve (GON). The trapezius fascia has been opened proximally, and a minimal amount of the medial portion of the semispinalis muscle has been removed to expose the body of the nerve. In this patient, the right greater occipital nerve (GON) looks flatter and more compressed than the left.

http://dx.doi.org/10.5772/66229

4.4. Rhinogenic triggers

In patients with weather-related migraines, and incomplete results from Botox injections, septonasal triggers should be considered. This pain is often described as behind the eye and can be unmasked after other primary sites are relieved either with surgery, BOTOX, or nerve blocks. A CT scan and nasal endoscopy are required to confirm diagnoses and will show any contact points and any complicated nasal pathology. Intranasal injection or spray of lidocaine may be used to further enhance the diagnostic power. At the time of surgery, local lidocaine and epinephrine are injected into the nose. Aroutine open or endoscopic septoplasty is used to address any contact points. In the cases of concha bullosa or significant enlargement of turbinates, full or partial resection of the turbinates is required. In cases of superior turbinate contact, outfracture or shaving is done and should only be performed by an expert plastic surgeon or ear-nose-throat surgeon experienced in this area.

Complications of this procedure include temporary or long-term nasal dryness. Synechiae and sinus infections are rare. Cerebrospinal fluid (CSF) leaks or more serious complications have not been reported in plastic surgery literature.

Routine activity within 1 week, and heavy activity within 3 weeks, is routine for all migraine surgery patients. Paresthesia and itching should improve with frequent massage and use of special brushes.

5. Conclusions

Select migraine headache patients, occipital neuralgia patients, and NDPH (New Daily Persistent Headache) patients can be successfully treated by surgical intervention. However, they should also be simultaneously seen by a neurologist, who can manage medications and rule out other diagnoses apart from migraine headache. Typically, these patients also have failed multiple classes of traditional conservative treatments. Careful documentation, such as patient migraine diaries, should be kept to track changes. Upon confirmation of migraine headache, various trigger sites can be identified by a constellation of symptoms and chemical denervation. Patients with severe anxiety and depression, medication overuse, and narcotic use respond poorly to surgery. Therefore, maximizing medical treatment by neurology following surgery is essential. Surgical decompression for treatment of migraine pain has proven significantly useful by multiple studies, both controlled prospective and retrospective [7].

Currently, surgical intervention becomes a viable option after complete exhaustion of other treatment methods. Rates of complication are low and potential benefits are life-changing. This small group of patients who do not respond to the available preventative and abortive treatments are often left with a very low quality of life. As a result, surgery is often the last resort for an effective treatment and potential permanent relief from their symptoms. In the future, further multicenter randomized prospective trials can elucidate which patients maybe better candidates and improve the response rate.

Author details

Michael Chung, Kyle Sanniec, Xingchen Li and Bardia Amirlak*

*Address all correspondence to: bardiaamirlak@gmail.com

UT Southwestern Department of Plastic Surgery, Dallas, TX, USA

References

[1] Stewart, W.F., et al., *Cumulative lifetime migraine incidence in women and men*. Cephalalgia, 2008. **28**(11): pp. 1170–8.

[2] Lipton, R.B., et al., *Migraine prevalence, disease burden, and the need for preventive therapy*. Neurology, 2007. **68**(5): pp. 343–9.

[3] Dodick, D.W., *Triptan nonresponder studies: implications for clinical practice*. Headache, 2005. **45**(2): pp. 156–62.

[4] Janis, J.E., et al., *A review of current evidence in the surgical treatment of migraine headaches*. Plast Reconstr Surg, 2014. **134**(4 Suppl 2): pp. 131S–41S.

[5] Singh, M., et al., *Causal relation between nerve compression and migraine symptoms and the therapeutic role of surgical decompression*. Plast Reconstr Surg Glob Open, 2015. **3**(5): p. e395.

[6] Dirnberger, F. and K. Becker, *Surgical treatment of migraine headaches by corrugator muscle resection*. Plast Reconstr Surg, 2004. **114**(3): pp. 652–7; discussion 658–9.

[7] Ducic, I., J.M. Felder, 3rd, and S.A. Fantus, *A systematic review of peripheral nerve interventional treatments for chronic headaches*. Ann Plast Surg, 2014. **72**(4): pp. 439–45.

[8] Guyuron, B., et al., *Comprehensive surgical treatment of migraine headaches*. Plast Reconstr Surg, 2005. **115**(1): pp. 1–9.

[9] Guyuron, B., et al., *Five-year outcome of surgical treatment of migraine headaches*. Plast Reconstr Surg, 2011. **127**(2): pp. 603–8.

[10] Janis, J.E., A. Dhanik, and J.H. Howard, *Validation of the peripheral trigger point theory of migraine headaches: single-surgeon experience using botulinum toxin and surgical decompression*. Plast Reconstr Surg, 2011. **128**(1): pp. 123–31.

[11] Poggi, J.T., B.E. Grizzell, and S.D. Helmer, *Confirmation of surgical decompression to relieve migraine headaches*. Plast Reconstr Surg, 2008. **122**(1): pp. 115–22; discussion 123–4.

[12] Goetz, C.G., *Textbook of clinical neurology*. 3rd ed. 2007, Philadelphia: Saunders Elsevier. xvii, 1364 p.

[13] Moskowitz, M.A., *The neurobiology of vascular head pain*. Ann Neurol, 1984. **16**(2): pp. 157–68.

[14] Welch, K.M., *Contemporary concepts of migraine pathogenesis*. Neurology, 2003. **61**(8 Suppl 4): p. S2–8.

[15] Guyuron, B., et al., *Electron microscopic and proteomic comparison of terminal branches of the trigeminal nerve in patients with and without migraine headaches*. Plast Reconstr Surg, 2014. **134**(5): pp. 796e–805e.

[16] Guyuron, B., et al., *Corrugator supercilii muscle resection and migraine headaches*. Plast Reconstr Surg, 2000. **106**(2): pp. 429–34; discussion 435–7.

[17] Becker, D. and B. Amirlak, *Beyond beauty: onobotulinumtoxinA (Botox(R)) and the management of migraine headaches*. Anesth Pain Med, 2012. **2**(1): pp. 5–11.

[18] Binder, W.J., et al., *Botulinum toxin type A (BOTOX) for treatment of migraine headaches: an open-label study*. Otolaryngol Head Neck Surg, 2000. **123**(6): pp. 669–76.

[19] Whitcup, S.M., et al., *Development of onabotulinumtoxinA for chronic migraine*. Ann N Y Acad Sci, 2014. **1329**: pp. 67–80.

[20] Dandy, W.E., *Treatment of hemicrania (migraine) by removal of the inferior cervical and first thoracic sympathetic ganglion*. Johns Hopkins Univ Bull, 1931. 48: pp. 357–361.

[21] Gardner, W.J., A. Stowell, and R. Dutlinger, *Resection of the greater superficial petrosal nerve in the treatment of unilateral headache*. J Neurosurg, 1947. **4**(2): pp. 105–14.

[22] Murillo, C.A., *Resection of the temporal neurovascular bundle for control of migraine headache*. Headache, 1968. **8**(3): pp. 112–7.

[23] Murphy, J.P., *Occipital neurectomy in the treatment of headache. Results in 30 cases*. Md State Med J, 1969. **18**(6): pp. 62–6.

[24] Guyuron, B., T. Tucker, and J. Davis, *Surgical treatment of migraine headaches*. Plast Reconstr Surg, 2002. **109**(7): pp. 2183–9.

[25] Guyuron, B., et al., *A placebo-controlled surgical trial of the treatment of migraine headaches*. Plast Reconstr Surg, 2009. **124**(2): pp. 461–8.

[26] Adenuga, P., et al., *Impact of preoperative narcotic use on outcomes in migraine surgery*. Plast Reconstr Surg, 2014. **134**(1): pp. 113–9.

[27] Gfrerer, L., et al., *Nonendoscopic deactivation of nerve triggers in migraine headache patients: surgical technique and outcomes*. Plast Reconstr Surg, 2014. **134**(4): pp. 771–8.

[28] Liu, M.T., H. Chim, and B. Guyuron, *Outcome comparison of endoscopic and transpalpebral decompression for treatment of frontal migraine headaches*. Plast Reconstr Surg, 2012. **129**(5): pp. 1113–9.

[29] Oturai, A.B., et al., *Neurosurgery for trigeminal neuralgia: comparison of alcohol block, neurectomy, and radiofrequency coagulation*. Clin J Pain, 1996. **12**(4): pp. 311–5.

[30] Taha, J.M. and J.M. Tew, Jr., *Comparison of surgical treatments for trigeminal neuralgia: reevaluation of radiofrequency rhizotomy*. Neurosurgery, 1996. **38**(5): pp. 865–71.

[31] Mathew, P.G., *A critical evaluation of migraine trigger site deactivation surgery*. Headache, 2014. **54**(1): pp. 142–52.

[32] Guyuron, B., *A discussion of "critical evaluation of migraine trigger site decompression surgery"*. Headache, 2014. **54**(6): pp. 1065–72.

[33] Guyuron, B., D. Harvey, and D. Reed, *A prospective randomized outcomes comparison of two temple migraine trigger site deactivation techniques*. Plast Reconstr Surg, 2015. **136**(1): pp. 159-65.

[34] Amirlak, B., et al., *The Anatomical Regional Targeted (ART) BOTOX injection technique. A new injection paradigm for the treatment of chronic headaches and migraines*. Plast Reconstr Surg Glob Open, *In Press* 2016.

[35] Liu, M.T., B.S. Armijo, and B. Guyuron, *A comparison of outcome of surgical treatment of migraine headaches using a constellation of symptoms versus botulinum toxin type A to identify the trigger sites*. Plast Reconstr Surg, 2012. **129**(2): pp. 413–9.

[36] Guyuron B, B.D., *Plastic Surgery: Indications and Practice*. Surgical management of migraine headaches, ed. T.T. Guyuron B, Davis J. 2008: Saunders: Elsevier, Health Sciences Division.

[37] Totonchi, A., N. Pashmini, and B. Guyuron, *The zygomaticotemporal branch of the trigeminal nerve: an anatomical study*. Plast Reconstr Surg, 2005. **115**(1): pp. 273–7.

[38] Sanniec, K., E. Borsting, and B. Amirlak, *Decompression-avulsion of the auriculotemporal nerve for treatment of migraines and chronic headaches*. Plast Reconstr Surg Glob Open, 2016. **4**(4): p. e678.

[39] Lee, M., et al., *The role of the third occipital nerve in surgical treatment of occipital migraine headaches*. J Plast Reconstr Aesthet Surg, 2013. **66**(10): pp. 1335–9.

Chapter 8

Management of Migraine Headaches: OnabotulinumtoxinA Injection

Michael Chung, Xingchen Li, Kyle Sanniec and Bardia Amirlak

Additional information is available at the end of the chapter

http://dx.doi.org/10.5772/67308

Abstract

Chronic migraines are a common debilitating headache disorder. Recently, there has been increasing interest in the use of onabotulinumtoxinA as a preventative treatment, as studies have shown significant benefits. In line with current accepted theories on the pathophysiology of migraines, the toxin works by both direct and indirect means to prevent peripheral and central nerve sensitization. While efficacy has been established, the technique for extracranial delivery of onabotulinumtoxinA continues to see changes in an effort to seek better outcomes. The PREEMPT injection protocol is the original injection paradigm design targeting broad muscle groups. The ART injection paradigm offers the ability to deliver onabotulinumtoxinA closer to culprit nerves, thus increasing its effect and also decreasing adverse effects. OnabotulinumtoxinA is an effective and well-tolerated option for selective patients seeking relief from migraine headaches.

Keywords: BTX, onabotulinum toxin, migraine, ART, PREEMPT, trigger site theory

1. Introduction

Chronic migraines are the most common type of headache in patients that seek treatment, according to the data compiled from several specialty headache centers in the United States [1–3]. It is a debilitating disorder that not only has the ability to severely reduce the quality of life, but also causes a heavy economic burden. However, among the high number of patients that suffer from chronic migraines, only a third receive prophylactic treatments [4].

Over the last couple of decades, there has been an increasing interest in the use of onabotulinumtoxinA (BTX-A) as a preventative treatment for migraine headaches. Over time, a number of well-designed large-scale studies demonstrated that this neurotoxin to be effective in reducing several measures of migraine symptomology [5–11]. The first major landmark study, called the PREEMPT (Phase III Research Evaluating Migraine Prophylaxis Therapy) trials, indicated that BTX-A is indeed effective and safe in treating migraine headaches. These studies showed a statistically significant reduction in the primary endpoint of headache day frequency in chronic migraine patients. They also demonstrated significant reductions in several other measures of migraine symptomology such as cumulative hours of headaches, headache days, and days of moderate/severe headaches [9]. Further studies indicated efficacy in reducing disease burden based on patient quality of life questionnaires [10, 11]. However, studies evaluating the effect of BTX-A on episodic migraines so far have not shown significant benefits [12–15]. This led to BTX-A being approved by the Food and Drug Administration (FDA) for the treatment of chronic migraine headaches. The injection paradigm used in the PREEMPT trails was designed based on the initial injection sites reported in earlier phase II trials [16, 17]. While the PREEMPT injection protocol is proven to be effective, research is ongoing with several other BTX-A injection techniques that have been developed. One in particular is the targeted approach, which was first done to pre-screen surgical decompression and later developed into a more formal technique used solely for preventative treatment purposes.

Currently, BTX-A is used to provide safe and effective long-term treatment for chronic migraine headaches. To appreciate the differences and advantages in BTX-A injection techniques between the two specialties, it is important to understand the different targets of injection, the trigger point and nerve compression hypothesis, mechanism of action of BTX-A in the treatment of migraines, and the anatomy of various muscles and nerves has only recently been elucidated by studies done between Cleveland and Dallas [6, 7, 18–20]. In this chapter, we discuss the PREEMPT injection paradigm and the Anatomical Regional Targeted (ART) BTX-A paradigm.

2. Mechanism of onabotulinumtoxinA

OnabotulinumtoxinA, one of the seven serotypes secreted by the *Clostridium botulinum* bacteria, is currently approved for use in several conditions including strabismus, blepharospasm, cervical dystonia, and glabellar lines. Only serotypes A and B are used in the medical context. The toxin works by blocking various activities at neuron junctions that depend on intracellular vesicle trafficking to the membrane, such as neurotransmitter release [21, 22]. Normally, stored acetylcholine is transmitted via intracellular vesicles that fuse at the surface outer membrane. OnabotulinumtoxinA cleaves the SNAP-25 protein at the surface membrane, inhibiting the SNARE complex system of vesicular fusion and thus preventing subsequent neurotransmitter release into the nerve junction [23]. In the context of pure cosmetic treatments, this mechanism inhibits contractions of superficial musculature on the face, eliminating the folding of skin. In the context of migraine treatment, the toxin likely works by inhibiting both motor and sensory neurons. Similar to cosmetic treatment, motor neuron inhibition is beneficial to the migraine patient. If nerve irritation is caused by impingement from an overactive muscle, the myorelaxant effect would reduce this irritation. On the other hand, another mechanism of migraine headaches genesis is hypersensitivity of sensory neurons, specifically nociceptor neurons. BTX-A acts as a direct analgesic by blocking these hyperexcitable nociceptors. Studies have shown that BTX-A blocks the release of a number of nociceptive mediators, preventing the hypersensitization of peripheral nociceptors [24]. By blocking peripheral pain signaling to the central nervous system, BTX-A thus indirectly blocks central sensitization. Additionally, BTX-A has direct effects on nerves. In animal studies, BTX-A has been shown to both prevent and reverse sensitization of nociceptors [25]. If given prophylactically, BTX-A reduces the increase in spontaneous firing rate caused by later sensitization. It also reduces the spontaneous firing rate of already sensitized nociceptors [25]. Due to inhibition of the SNARE complex, the activity of chemoreceptors (TRPA1 and TRPV1) required for nociception is also reduced [26]. Importantly, recent evidence suggests that depositing BTX-A closer to nerves increases its effect, versus being distributed within a muscle group [26]. Therefore, the toxin's benefit in the prophylactic treatment of chronic migraines is likely due to several interacting effects including the inhibition of overactive motor neurons and the prevention/reversal of nociceptor sensitization [27].

3. Diagnosis of chronic migraines and candidacy for onabotulinumtoxinA

Prior to being treated for migraine headaches by BTX-A injection, it is critical for the patient to be seen by a board-certified neurologist, preferably one who specializes in headache medicine. If the neurologist does not offer BTX-A injection, collaboration with other specialties such as plastic surgery, ENT, or pain management for the injections can be done. A multidisciplinary team approach with plastic surgery, neurology, psychiatry, sleep medicine, and pain management working in conjunction with each other is an effective and preferred approach. The neurologist should evaluate and confirm the diagnosis of chronic migraine headache, ruling out other likely causes of recurring headaches that may not respond to BTX-A injection. Results from the PREEMPT part 1 and part 2 trials established BTX-A as safe and effective for chronic migraine patients. However, BTX-A should be avoided in patients who have previous hypersensitivity reactions to the toxin. Other contraindications include pre-existing neuromuscular disorders (myasthenia gravis and Lambert-Eaton syndrome), peripheral motor neuropathies, and amyotrophic lateral sclerosis that can increase the risk of significant side effects. It is unclear how effective BTX-A is in treating other commonly seen headache types, such as cluster, tension, and episodic headaches, as results have been mixed [15–17, 28–30]. Lastly, the majority of insurance carriers in the United States require documentation of migraine and headaches days, and previous failure of several classes of migraine medications.

4. Trigger sites and peripheral nerve irritation hypothesis

Because of its complex and multifactorial etiology, the exact pathophysiology of migraine headaches has yet to be completely elucidated. There are several commonly accepted theories based on central and peripheral mechanisms. In the context of onabotulinumtoxinA injection for migraine headaches, local inflammation sensitizes sensory neurons and upregulates the recruitment of sensory nociceptors [31–38]. As alluded to earlier, migraine pathophysiology involves irritation of peripheral nerves. Specifically, it involves several branches of the trigeminal nerve. Subsequent repeated irritation of the nerve causes an augmented perception of pain. The trigger point hypothesis attempts to explain this cycle of inflammation and trigeminal neuronal hypersensitivity. It takes into account that patients are often able to describe the origin of their migraine pain in a specific area, and that each site of origin leads to a different constellation of symptoms. Among other mechanisms, irritation of extracranial nerves in the periphery can be caused by overactivity of surrounding musculature, tight fascial bands, and intimate neurovascular relationships. Therefore, irritation of peripheral nerves by adjacent muscular contraction or other contact points can cause release of inflammatory factors, triggering the onset of migraine headaches. In this context, onabotulinumtoxinA can be targeted to these potential trigger sites in an attempt to prevent or inhibit the inflammatory cycle leading to peripheral and central sensitization. This theory and its implication in the success or failure of migraine surgery should not influence the fact that anatomical knowledge of the nerve locations can improve BTX-A injection techniques. Even if some neurologists do not hold the peripheral nerve compression theory correct, evidence now shows that BTX-A is most effective when deposited closer to nerves, acting by means of either direct reduction of chemoreceptors on the nociceptor membrane surface, or indirect decrease in activity by reducing mechanosensitivity [25, 26].

Trigger sites are identified by regions where the pain originates, rather than other final locations where the pain may travel. To assess which sites are active, a Migraine Diary should be completed by patients each day for at least 4 weeks. Since patients often do not pay especially close attention to the exact location where pain begins, this log is very useful in keeping track of trigger origin sites. In addition to the migraine diary, a thorough history should be obtained to differentiate between sites where pain begins and sites where pain may radiate to. Because trigger sites are where the pain originates, injection of targeted BTX-A should be focused in these sites and not where the pain ends. However, a more liberal approach to targeted injection is to inject all the regions. Currently, there are six major trigger sites relevant to available treatment methods, which can be categorized into several "regions": frontal (Site I), temporal (Site II), rhinogenic (Site III), occipital (Sites IV and VI), and auriculotemporal (Site V). **Site I** refers to headaches beginning in the lateral and central forehead areas, with central and cephalad radiation. Patients often describe the pain beginning above the eye and moving from outside to inside. At times, palpation with a single finger at the area of the supraorbital and supratrochlear nerve will reveal tender areas where the supraorbital nerve (SON) and supratrochlear nerve (STN) are involved. In some cases, hypertrophy of the corrugator supercilii muscle may be visible on physical exam. **Site II**, or the temporal trigger site, is associated with headaches originating in the temple. Often times, pain radiates toward the lateral temporal and posterior auricular areas. The temporalis muscle may be larger than normal, or tighter than usual. However, it is important to differentiate temporomandibular joint (TMJ) pathology, as it is not a trigger site for migraine headaches. In this region, the zygomaticotemporal branch of the trigeminal nerve (ZTBTN) is involved in the generation of pain. **Site III** refers to pain of nasoseptal origin. This pain is usually associated with weather changes and atmospheric pressure changes, usually beginning in the early hours of the morning. Patients may complain of rhinitis, hyposmia, anosmia, halitosis, and dental pain. Because of this, they can also complain of breathing problems. In addition, this pain is generally described as starting behind the eye and radiating outward. Oxymetazoline nasal spray is used to temporarily abort headaches originating from this site. Of note, septal triggers should be considered if pain persists despite BTX-A injection in other trigger sites. To confirm an active trigger site in the septal area, imaging via computed tomography scan is required. Intranasal pathology such as septal deviation contacting turbinates, concha bullosae, and other masses can be identified and surgically treated. It is important to rule out septonasal origin, as BTX-A generally does not improve pain originating from site III. **Site IV** occipital trigger site refers to headaches originating in the back of the neck and radiating anteriorly. This area usually correlates with the anatomical course of the greater occipital nerve (GON). Palpation in this area usually reveals a point of maximal tenderness that corresponds to the location where the nerve pierces the semispinalis capitis muscle. Some injection techniques target the semispinalis and splenius capitis, as well as the occipitalis muscle, but generally BTX-A is deposited as close to the nerve as possible. Patients may also complain of retroauricular pain associated with this site. Of note, it is possible that an intimate neurovascular relationship between the greater occipital nerve and occipital artery at this trigger site plays a major role in migraine development [6, 18, 20, 39]. The close relationship of the greater occipital nerve with the occipital artery can cause pain to fluctuate with weather, as arterial vascular tone changes. In general, pain in the occipital region mostly involves the GON, while the third occipital nerve (TON) may be involved to a lesser degree. **Site V** refers to pain in the area corresponding to the auriculotemporal nerve (AT). Pain in this area is caused by TMJ facial bands inferiorly and the temporal artery more superiorly, causing irritation to the AT nerve [40]. Finally, **Site VI** refers to the area around the lesser occipital nerve.

While these areas are the major sites relevant to currently available treatment modalities, a number of other sites have been reported to cause significant pain. The trapezius muscle group, TMJ muscle group, sternocleidomastoid muscle, and masseter are few examples. While patient description should aid in the selection and specific location of injection sites, actual injection is based on the anatomy of the culprit nerves and surrounding tissue.

5. Techniques for injection

5.1. PREEMPT injection paradigm [24]

The injection protocol used in the phase III PREEMPT trials were based on, and developed upon, earlier phase II studies that demonstrated safety and efficacy in the use of onabotulinum toxin for chronic migraine patients. Using this PREEMPT injection paradigm, the phase III part 1 and part 2 studies confirmed significant reduction in the frequency of headache days and low rates of adverse events [9, 41]. At 24 weeks, pooled data from both trials reported a significant difference in the reduction of headache days compared to placebo. Specifically, those who underwent 24 weeks of BTX-A injection had a 7.4 day reduction, while placebo had a 4.7 reduction in headache days [10]. Thus, the PREEMPT injection protocol is a proven prophylactic treatment for chronic migraine patients.

As the first formal injection protocol described, the PREEMPT technique is a combination of a "fixed site" and "follow the pain" approaches. This was based on a number of earlier studies employing different approaches. From these studies, this combination approach was determined as the most optimal protocol to be used in the PREEMPT trials [24]. A total of 155 units are injected into 31 fixed sites, targeting a number of muscle groups. In addition to these fixed site and fixed dose (FSFD) sites, an additional eight sites and 40 units can be injected according to physician discernment in a "follow the pain" approach. Therefore, the PREEMPT injection paradigm uses a minimum of 155 units and a maximum of 195 units, which corresponds well with the determined optimal dosage range between 150 and 200 units [24]. **Figure 1** shows the PREEMPT injection protocol in each area. A standard 30-gauge 0.5-inch syringe is used, and an injection interval of 12 weeks is followed.

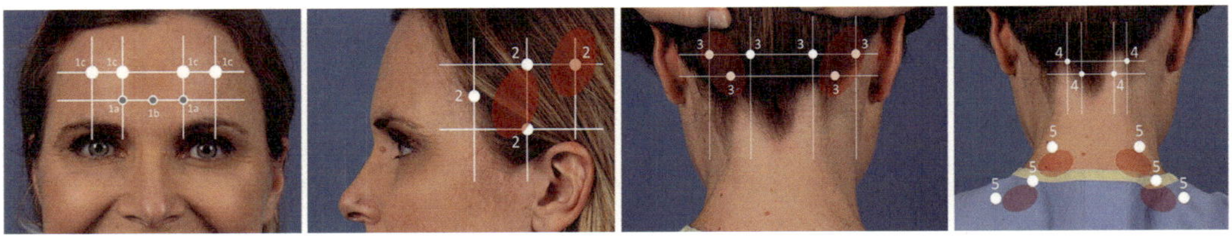

Figure 1. PREEMPT injection protocol. Locations of fixed site, fixed dose injections: (1a) procerus, (1b) corrugators, (1c) frontalis, (2) temporalis, (3) occipitalis, (4) cervical paraspinal, and (5) trapezius muscle. Follow-the-pain injection areas are indicated in red color.

5.1.1. Frontal

In the frontal region, a total of 35 units are injected in a shallow manner into four muscle groups. First, the corrugator muscle is injected bilaterally 1.5 cm above the medial superior edge of the orbital ridge, with 10 units into each side. In the midline, the procerus is injected with 5 units in a location midway between the two corrugator injections. Finally, injection of the frontalis is divided into four sites, with 20 units total. On one side, the medial injection is 1.5 cm above the corrugator injection, and the lateral injection is 1.5 cm away from the medial injection in the same horizontal plane. This is repeated on the opposite side of the forehead.

5.1.2. Temporal

In the temporal region, the temporalis muscle is the main muscle group targeted. Injection in this area consists of four sites on each side of the head. A total of 20 units are injected into each side. The first injection is behind the anterior border of the temporalis muscle. The second injection is 0.5 cm above and 1.5 cm posterior to the first injection. The third and fourth injection is 0.5 cm posterior and inferior to the second injection, respectively. This is repeated on the opposite side. As mentioned earlier, additional units can be injected on both or just one side, and is based on palpation for significant tenderness and pain that requires additional treatment.

5.1.3. Occipital

The occipitalis muscle group is injected with 15 units in three sites on each side, totaling 30 units. The first injection is 1 cm lateral to and above the occipital protuberance. The second injection is given 1 cm lateral and 1 cm above the first injection. Finally, the third injection is 1 cm medial and 1 cm above the first injection. Similar to the temple area injection, physicians can follow the pain by palpating for significant areas of tenderness, and inject additional units.

5.1.4. Cervical spine and paraspinal muscle groups

In the area of the back of the neck, the PREEMPT protocol targets the semispinalis and splenius muscle groups. Injection consists of two sites on each side with 20 units total. On each side, the first injection is 3–5 cm inferior and just lateral to the occipital protuberance. Another injection is made 1 cm superior and lateral to the first.

5.1.5. Trapezius

The trapezius muscle is injected superiorly into three sites on each side, with 30 units total. The fixed dose is 5 units into each of the six total sites. One injection is made into the lateral portion of the muscle, another to the middle aspect, and one medially and superior within the medial portion of the muscle. With results from palpation for tenderness and pain, the physician can inject additional sites within the muscle group.

5.2. ART injection technique: Anatomical, Regional, and Targeted [42]

While the PREEMPT trials and its associated injection paradigm have paved the way for the development of BTX-A injection in migraine headaches, several other injection techniques have been developed, including the Anatomical, Regional, and Targeted (ART) injection paradigm. In contrast to the "fixed site" and "follow the pain" approach of the PREEMPT protocol, the ART technique offers a dynamic injection paradigm based on anatomical studies and surgical experiences in the decompression of nerves [42].

The ART injection paradigm can be described as Anatomical, Regional, and Targeted [42]. In this approach, injection is not necessarily targeted to a broad muscle group. Rather, this injection paradigm is designed based more on the *direct* effects of onabotulinum toxin on peripheral nerves, which have been previously described [25, 26, 43, 44]. As a result, injections rely heavily on accurate understanding of nerve anatomy and delivery of the toxin as close to the nerve as possible. The term "Anatomical" refers to injections based on the accurate location and depth of a nerve, and its surrounding musculature. "Regional" refers to focused injections at regions where pain originates (frontal, temporal, or occipital). "Targeted" refers to injections based on the topography of tender areas, which may not always correspond with known anatomical compression points. Therefore, the ART injection approach has the potential to be more individualized to each patient's unique picture of migraine pain.

While the PREEMPT injection paradigm dictates the exact dosage delivered to each site, the ART injection protocol is less strict on how much is injected. Previous studies have showed the optimal dosage range per injection cycle is between 150 and 200 units [24]. The standard ART dosage consists of 155 units delivered across several sites: 45 units into the frontal site, 25 units into the temples, 50 units to the GON, 10 units to the LON, 15 units split into the tails of the GON and LON, 5 units in the area of the AT nerve, and finally 5 units in the area of the tail of the AT nerve. This standard is the injection pattern given to patients who report pain in all trigger sites. However, upon physician discretion, more units can be delivered to certain areas, or none in certain trigger sites, according to what the patient reports.

5.2.1. Site I: Frontal

In Site I, injection of BTX-A is based on irritation of the supraorbital and supratrochlear nerves (SON and STN). In this site, the injection is more anatomical than targeted. If BTX-A is injected in areas of maximal tenderness here closer to the orbital rim, the risk for lid ptosis and diplopia is high. Therefore, injection is more fixed in this area. The corrugator supercilii muscle (CSM) is thought to compress the SON and STN, but any of the other glabellar muscles has the potential to as well (procerus, depressor supercilii). In addition, fibrous bands in the supraorbital foramen, or a boney foramen, could also be sources for proximal compression and pain. Before injecting into this area, the topographical anatomy of the corrugator muscle can be clearly visualized by asking the patient to frown. Of note, studies in plastic surgery literature have further outlined the anatomy of the corrugator, which is not followed accurately in the PREEMPT/Allergan injection protocol (**Figure 2**). The CSM begins 3 mm lateral to the midline and extends 43 mm laterally. Superiorly, it extends 33 mm from the pupil. An ice pack is used to cool the area before injection, as it is important to reduce anxiety and pain in the migraine patient. Digital occlusion of the supraorbital and supratrochlear vessels with the non-dominant thumb reduces the risk of "microhematomas". A short 0.5 inch 30-gauge needle with 0.1 cc graduation is used to inject 12.5 units into each side with a five-point standard injection (**Figure 3**). Based on correct anatomy, injection should be deeper medially and more superficial laterally. Single injections can be done on each side using a longer needle inserted superficially on the lateral side and extended deeply toward the medial side. Injection should be done as the needle is advancing, as it provides for the best control. If bleeding is present, gauze can be used, but it is critical not to press with excess pressure as the toxin can diffuse into unwanted areas in the upper lid.

Injection into the frontalis muscle should be only in the upper half of the forehead (**Figure 3**). Injecting lower on the forehead leads to a higher rate of lid ptosis. A total of 15–20 units is injected. This injection not only targets the distal portions of the SON and STN, but relaxation of the frontalis muscle reduces cephalic pull that can cause tension in the proximal nerve areas.

5.2.2. Site II: Temporal

Injection into the temporal area is again more anatomical than targeted. The zygomaticotemporal branch of the trigeminal nerve (ZTBTN) emerges approximately 17 mm posterolateral and 6.5 mm cephalad to the lateral canthus. This point of exit from the temporalis muscle is seen consistently in cadaver studies [45]. A long 30-gauge needle should pierce the temporalis muscle 1 cm posterolateral to this point to deposit 12.5 units on each side (**Figure 4**). The injection should be fanned deeply in a 1.5 cm radius. Additionally, a single deep injection at the point of nerve exit over the deep temporal fascia should also be performed.

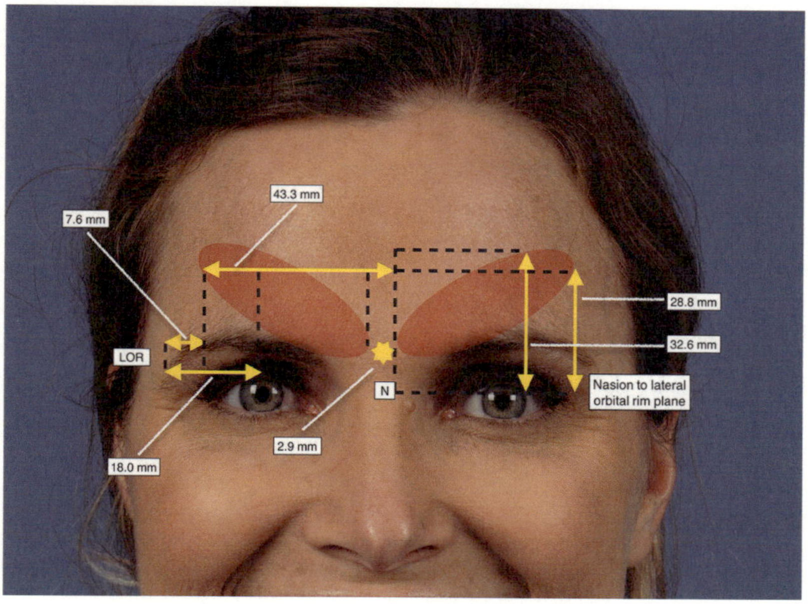

Figure 2. The location of the corrugator muscle.

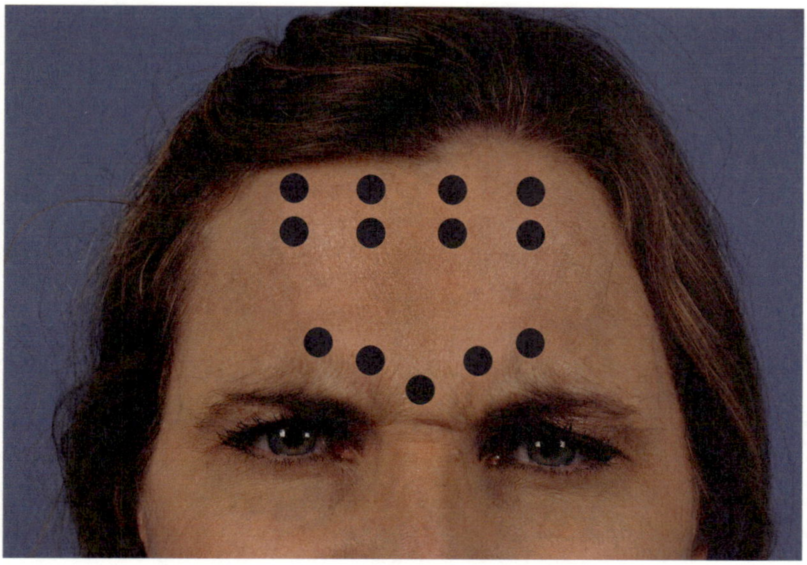

Figure 3. ART frontal trigger site injection. Image demonstrating injection sites over the corrugator muscle. The patient frowns to assist in finding the correct locations. The SON and STN nerves are targeted here, as well as the frontalis muscle.

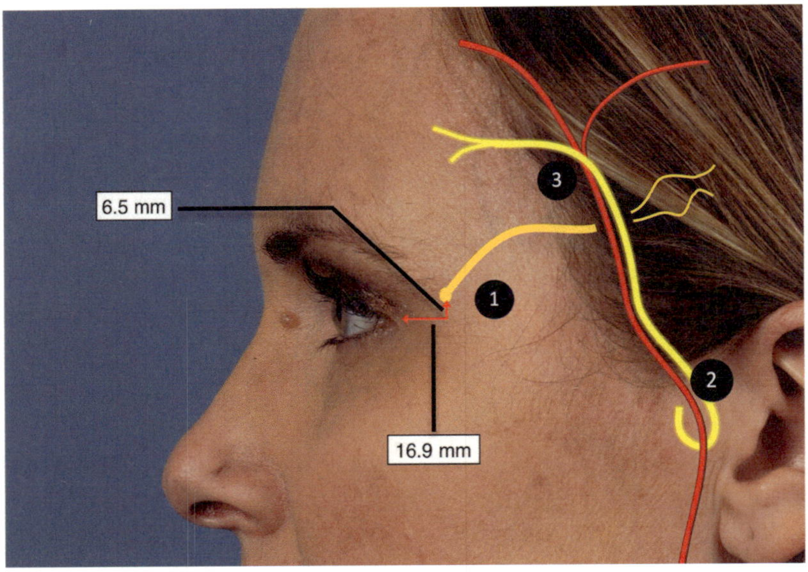

Figure 4. ART temporal trigger site injections. Figure demonstrating the relationship between the auriculotemporal nerve (AT), zygomaticotemporal nerve (ZTBTN), and the superficial temporal artery. It is important to note that the ZTBTN is on a different fascial plane, and does not normally contact the AT nerve or temporal artery. Injection sites include: (1) 1.5 cm posterolateral emergence of ZTBTN from deep temporal fascia. (2) fascial band compression at proximal AT. (3) Distal AT area corresponding to crossing with the superficial temporal artery.

The auriculotemporal nerve (AT) is another potential source of nerve irritation in the temporal area. This nerve is referred to as **Site V**. Injection at this site is more targeted than anatomical. BTX-A delivery should be guided by the patient's descriptions of tender areas, which may not always correspond with areas of anatomical compression. Injections should be in two sites: one near the proximal AT area where fibrous bands can compress the nerve, and one near the distal AT where it crosses the superficial temporal artery [42] (**Figure 4**).

5.2.3. Site III: Nasoseptal

BTX-A cannot be delivered to this area. A computed tomography scan should be done to elucidate areas of turbinate contact or other masses. Currently, the only treatment for this site is surgical correction.

5.2.4. Site IV: Occipital

Injection in Site IV is based on irritation of the occipital nerves: greater occipital nerve (GON), lesser occipital nerve (LON), and the third occipital nerve (TON). Although the LON can be referred to as **Site VI**, its treatment is considered together with other occipital sites. The GON is most commonly the primary site of pain. This injection is both targeted and anatomical. The nerve consistently pierces the semispinalis capitis muscle at a point 1.5 cm lateral to the midline and 3 cm below to the occipital protuberance (**Figure 5**). However, the area of maximal tenderness is often 0.5–1 cm lateral to this point. Therefore, BTX-A injection should be targeted to this area. When injecting this nerve, it is critical to inject deeply enough to pierce the trapezius fascia, where the nerve resides. A sturdier 27-gauge long needle is used to ensure penetration of the thick fascia, with 25 units injected into each side. The LON is injected similarly in a targeted and anatomical approach, using 10 units total for both sides (**Figure 5**). The point of maximal tenderness often corresponds anatomically within 0.5 cm of the emergence of the LON behind the sternocleidomastoid muscle [46]. The LON emerges 6.4 cm lateral to the posterior midline drawn through cervical spine, and 7.5 cm caudal from a horizontal line drawn between the most superolateral aspects of the external auditory canals [47]. Additionally, patients sometimes describe pain in the areas corresponding to the distal tails of the GON and LON. In these areas, terminal branches of the occipital artery intertwine with the occipital nerves.

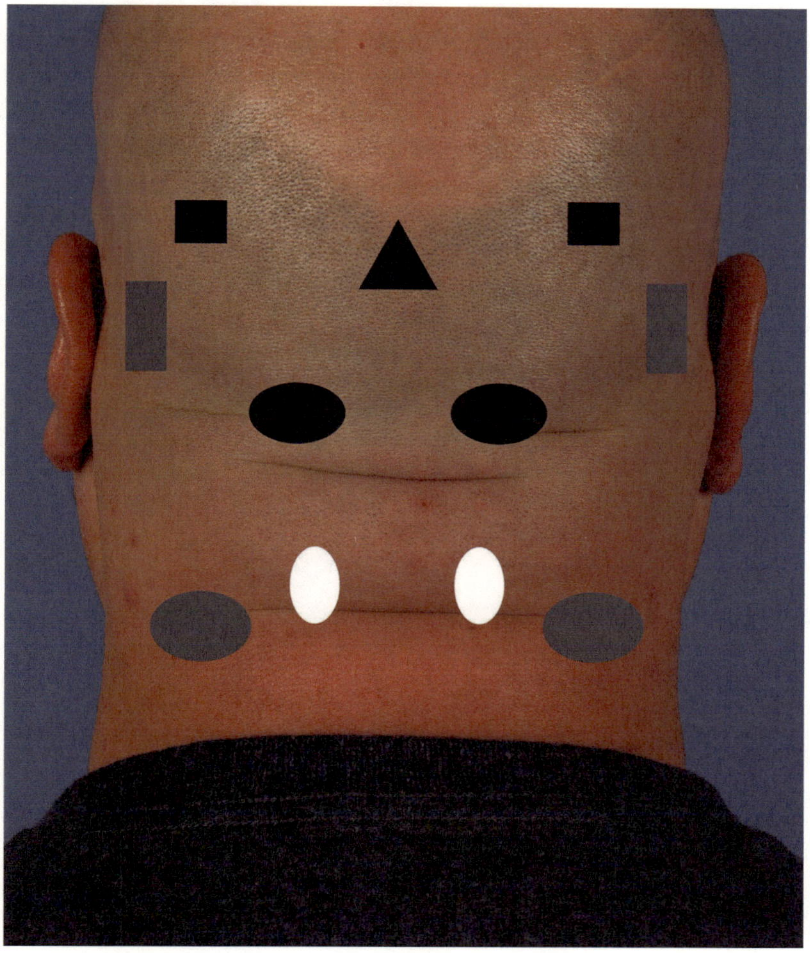

Figure 5. ART occipital trigger site injection sites and landmarks. Occipital protuberance (triangle), GON (black oval), tail of GON (black square), LON (gray oval), tail of LON (gray square), 3rd occipital nerve (white circle).

6. Conclusion

OnabotulinumtoxinA injection is an effective strategy to treat chronic migraine. At 56 weeks, the percentage of patients in the PREEMPT trials that received at least 50% reduction in headache days was 68%, significantly better than the reduction seen in patients who received placebo [48]. In addition to being effective, BTX-A has also been shown to cause very minimal adverse effects. Some commonly seen complications include neck pain/weakness, eyelid ptosis, and injection site pain. There have been no reported deaths among migraine BTX-A studies, and only 1.4–3.8% of patients discontinued treatment due to adverse effects [9, 10, 16, 17, 24].

BTX-A injection is an effective and well-tolerated treatment option for chronic migraine patients who have previously failed a number of traditional medications. It is most effective in patients who suffer from a higher frequency of headache days, such as those seen in chronic migraines. Additionally, it is well known that chronic migraine patients often suffer from medication overuse. In a subanalysis of PREEMPT trial results, BTX-A demonstrated significant effectiveness in reducing frequency of headache days even in patients who are designated with medication overuse [49]. Sometimes, patients may not respond from the first injection interval. It has been shown even among patients that fail to respond initially, a meaningful proportion of patients responded in the second and third treatment cycles [50]. ART injection on the other hand is a newer, expanded, and more refined version of the targeted injection based on recent neurology data and theories suggesting that BTX-A is more effective if deposited closer to nerves. Although available studies are less robust, preliminary clinical results show less complications than PREEMPT.

While onabotulinumtoxinA injection has been shown to be both safe and effective among a broad group of patients, demonstrating versatile and robust efficacy, research is ongoing to develop the best and most efficient ways to deliver this treatment. Knowledge of potential culprit nerves and the accurate understanding of surrounding tissue anatomy are essential to maximize efficacy and efficiency in chronic migraine pain management.

Author details

Michael Chung, Xingchen Li, Kyle Sanniec and Bardia Amirlak*

*Address all correspondence to: Bardia.Amirlak@UTSouthwestern.edu

UT Southwestern Department of Plastic Surgery, Dallas, Texas, USA

References

[1] Headache Classification, C., et al., New appendix criteria open for a broader concept of chronic migraine. Cephalalgia, 2006. **26**(6): pp. 742–6.

[2] Pascual, J., Colas, R., and Castillo, J., Epidemiology of chronic daily headache. Current Pain and Headache Reports, 2001. **5**(6): pp. 529–36.

[3] Silberstein, S.D. and Lipton, R.B., Chronic daily headache. Current Opinion in Neurology, 2000. **13**(3): pp. 277–83.

[4] Bigal, M.E., et al., Chronic migraine in the population: Burden, diagnosis, and satisfaction with treatment. Neurology, 2008. **71**(8): pp. 559–66.

[5] Guyuron, B., et al., Corrugator supercilii muscle resection and migraine headaches. Plastic and Reconstructive Surgery, 2000. **106**(2): pp. 429–34; discussion 435–7.

[6] Mosser, S.W., et al., The anatomy of the greater occipital nerve: Implications for the etiology of migraine headaches. Plastic and Reconstructive Surgery, 2004. **113**(2): pp. 693–7; discussion 698–700.

[7] Totonchi, A., Pashmini, N., and Guyuron, B., The zygomaticotemporal branch of the trigeminal nerve: an anatomical study. Plastic and Reconstructive Surgery, 2005. **115**(1): pp. 273–7.

[8] Guyuron, B, Plastic surgery: Indications and practice. Surgical Management of Migraineheadaches, ed. T.T. Guyuron B, Davis J. Philadelphia, United States 2008: Saunders: Elsevier – Health Sciences Division.

[9] Aurora, S.K., et al., OnabotulinumtoxinA for treatment of chronic migraine: Results from the double-blind, randomized, placebo-controlled phase of the PREEMPT 1 trial. Cephalalgia, 2010. **30**(7): pp. 793–803.

[10] Dodick, D.W., et al., OnabotulinumtoxinA for treatment of chronic migraine: pooled results from the double-blind, randomized, placebo-controlled phases of the PREEMPT clinical program. Headache, 2010. **50**(6): pp. 921–36.

[11] Lipton, R.B., et al., OnabotulinumtoxinA improves quality of life and reduces impact of chronic migraine. Neurology, 2011. **77**(15): pp. 1465–72.

[12] Elkind, A.H., et al., A series of three sequential, randomized, controlled studies of repeated treatments with botulinum toxin type A for migraine prophylaxis. The Journal of Pain, 2006. **7**(10): pp. 688–96.

[13] Relja, M., et al., A multicentre, double-blind, randomized, placebo-controlled, parallel group study of multiple treatments of botulinum toxin type A (BoNTA) for the prophylaxis of episodic migraine headaches. Cephalalgia, 2007. **27**(6): pp. 492–503.

[14] Saper, J.R., et al., A double-blind, randomized, placebo-controlled comparison of botulinum toxin type a injection sites and doses in the prevention of episodic migraine. Pain Medicine, 2007. **8**(6): pp. 478–85.

[15] Silberstein, S., et al., Botulinum toxin type A as a migraine preventive treatment. For the BOTOX Migraine Clinical Research Group. Headache, 2000. **40**(6): pp. 445–50.

[16] Mathew, N.T., et al., Botulinum toxin type A (BOTOX) for the prophylactic treatment of chronic daily headache: A randomized, double-blind, placebo-controlled trial. Headache, 2005. **45**(4): pp. 293–307.

[17] Silberstein, S.D., et al., Botulinum toxin type A for the prophylactic treatment of chronic daily headache: A randomized, double-blind, placebo-controlled trial. Mayo Clinic Proceedings, 2005. **80**(9): pp. 1126–37.

[18] Caviggioli, F., et al., Neurovascular compression of the greater occipital nerve: Implications for migraine headaches. Plastic and Reconstructive Surgery, 2012. **129**(2): pp. 353e–4.

[19] Janis, J.E., et al., The anatomy of the corrugator supercilii muscle: Part II. Supraorbital nerve branching patterns. Plastic and Reconstructive Surgery, 2008. **121**(1): pp. 233–40.

[20] Shimizu, S., et al., Can proximity of the occipital artery to the greater occipital nerve act as a cause of idiopathic greater occipital neuralgia? An anatomical and histological evaluation of the artery-nerve relationship. Plastic and Reconstructive Surgery, 2007. **119**(7): pp. 2029–34; discussion 2035–6.

[21] Schiavo, G., Rossetto, O., and Montecucco, C., Clostridial neurotoxins as tools to investigate the molecular events of neurotransmitter release. Seminars in Cell Biology, 1994. **5**(4): pp. 221–9.

[22] Pearce, L.B., et al., Pharmacologic characterization of botulinum toxin for basic science and medicine. Toxicon, 1997. **35**(9): pp. 1373–412.

[23] Humeau, Y., et al., How botulinum and tetanus neurotoxins block neurotransmitter release. Biochimie, 2000. **82**(5): pp. 427–46.

[24] Blumenfeld, A., et al., Method of injection of onabotulinumtoxinA for chronic migraine: A safe, well-tolerated, and effective treatment paradigm based on the PREEMPT clinical program. Headache, 2010. **50**(9): pp. 1406–18.

[25] Burstein, R., et al., Selective inhibition of meningeal nociceptors by botulinum neurotoxin type A: Therapeutic implications for migraine and other pains. Cephalalgia, 2014. **34**(11): pp. 853–69.

[26] Zhang, X., et al., Extracranial injections of botulinum neurotoxin type A inhibit intracranial meningeal nociceptors' responses to stimulation of TRPV1 and TRPA1 channels: Are we getting closer to solving this puzzle? Cephalalgia, 2016. **36**(9): pp. 875–86.

[27] Durham, P.L. and Cady, R., Insights into the mechanism of onabotulinumtoxinA in chronic migraine. Headache, 2011. **51**(10): pp. 1573–7.

[28] Aurora, S.K., et al., Botulinum toxin type a prophylactic treatment of episodic migraine: A randomized, double-blind, placebo-controlled exploratory study. Headache, 2007. **47**(4): pp. 486–99.

[29] Freitag, F.G., et al., Botulinum toxin type A in the treatment of chronic migraine without medication overuse. Headache, 2008. **48**(2): pp. 201–9.

[30] Silberstein, S.D., et al., Botulinum toxin type A in the prophylactic treatment of chronic tension-type headache: A multicentre, double-blind, randomized, placebo-controlled, parallel-group study. Cephalalgia, 2006. **26**(7): pp. 790–800.

[31] Burstein, R., Collins, B., and Jakubowski, M., Defeating migraine pain with triptans: A race against the development of cutaneous allodynia. Annals of Neurology, 2004. **55**(1): pp. 19–26.

[32] Burstein, R., et al., An association between migraine and cutaneous allodynia. Annals of Neurology, 2000. **47**(5): pp. 614–24.

[33] de Tommaso, M., et al., The three responses of the blink reflex in adult and juvenile migraine. Acta Neurologica Belgica, 2000. **100**(2): pp. 96–102.

[34] Goetz, C.G., Textbook of Clinical Neurology. 3rd ed. 2007, Philadelphia: Saunders Elsevier. xvii, 1364 p.

[35] Grosser, K., et al., Olfactory and trigeminal event-related potentials in migraine. Cephalalgia, 2000. **20**(7): pp. 621–31.

[36] Moskowitz, M.A., The neurobiology of vascular head pain. Annals of Neurology, 1984. **16**(2): pp. 157–68.

[37] Welch, K.M., Contemporary concepts of migraine pathogenesis. Neurology, 2003. **61**(8 Suppl 4): pp. S2-8.

[38] Williamson, D.J. and R.J. Hargreaves, Neurogenic inflammation in the context of migraine. Microscopy Research and Technique, 2001. **53**(3): pp. 167–78.

[39] Janis, J.E., et al., Neurovascular compression of the greater occipital nerve: implications for migraine headaches. Plastic and Reconstructive Surgery, 2010. **126**(6): pp. 1996–2001.

[40] Sanniec, K., Borsting, E., and B. Amirlak, Decompression-avulsion of the auriculotemporal nerve for treatment of migraines and chronic headaches. Plastic and Reconstructive Surgery – Global Open, 2016. **4**(4): pp. e678.

[41] Diener, H.C., et al., OnabotulinumtoxinA for treatment of chronic migraine: Results from the double-blind, randomized, placebo-controlled phase of the PREEMPT 2 trial. Cephalalgia, 2010. **30**(7): pp. 804–14.

[42] Amirlak, B., et al., The Anatomical Regional Targeted (ART) BOTOX injection technique. A new injection paradigm for the treatment of chronic headaches and migraines. Plastic and Reconstructive Surgery – Global Open, *in press* 2016. DOI 10.1097/gox.0000000000001194

[43] Raddant, A.C. and Russo, A.F., Calcitonin gene-related peptide in migraine: Intersection of peripheral inflammation and central modulation. Expert Reviews in Molecular Medicine, 2011. **13**: pp. e36.

[44] Zhang, X., et al., Activation of central trigeminovascular neurons by cortical spreading depression. Annals of Neurology, 2011. **69**(5): pp. 855–65.

[45] Guyuron, B., et al., Five-year outcome of surgical treatment of migraine headaches. Plastic and Reconstructive Surgery, 2011. **127**(2): pp. 603–8.

[46] Guyuron, B., et al., A placebo-controlled surgical trial of the treatment of migraine headaches. Plastic and Reconstructive Surgery, 2009. **124**(2): pp. 461–8.

[47] Lee, M., et al., An anatomical study of the lesser occipital nerve and its potential compression points: Implications for surgical treatment of migraine headaches. Plastic and Reconstructive Surgery, 2013. **132**(6): pp. 1551–6.

[48] Aurora, S.K., et al., OnabotulinumtoxinA for treatment of chronic migraine: pooled analyses of the 56-week PREEMPT clinical program. Headache, 2011. **51**(9): pp. 1358–73.

[49] Silberstein, S.D., et al., OnabotulinumtoxinA for treatment of chronic migraine: PREEMPT 24-week pooled subgroup analysis of patients who had acute headache medication overuse at baseline. Journal of the Neurological Sciences, 2013. **331**(1–2): pp. 48–56.

[50] Silberstein, S.D., et al., Per cent of patients with chronic migraine who responded per onabotulinumtoxinA treatment cycle: PREEMPT. Journal of Neurology, Neurosurgery, and Psychiatry, 2015. **86**(9): pp. 996–1001.

Chapter 9

Acupuncture as a Therapy for Headache

Sumire Chiku and Yasushi Shibata

Additional information is available at the end of the chapter

http://dx.doi.org/10.5772/65012

Abstract

Acupuncture has been used to treat various diseases, and there are many reports from various countries around the world as a therapy for headaches. Acupuncture has been used to relieve tension-type headaches and prevent migraine attacks. In patients with migraine without aura, the number of headache attacks and analgesic use among patients who received acupuncture was significantly decreased compared to those who were treated with flunarizine. However, few articles have classified headaches in detail and examined the effectiveness of acupuncture. Thus, there is no clear evidence of the types of headache for which acupuncture is effective or whether acupuncture should be performed in the attack phase or intermittent phase. Functional MRI (fMRI) is a form of objective imaging study. Recently, a study was performed to investigate brain dysfunction in patients with migraine and chronic tension-type headache. In the study of the pain-induced activation of fMRI, migraine patients demonstrated specific brain activation in the interictal period compared to controls. We hypothesize that acupuncture affects not only peripheral circulation, but also central nervous function. However, few scientific studies have investigated the effects of acupuncture for headache by assessing cerebral function.

Keywords: headache, acupuncture, acupoint, tension-type headache, migraine

1. Introduction

Headache is prevalent worldwide and was reported as the sixth most frequent global cause of years lived with disability in 2013 [1]. When limited to migraine, its frequency is 19th place, and when limited to women, its frequency is 12th place [2]. The prevalence rate of tension-type headache is also high, and it was reported to be 38% in worldwide [3]. However, the diagnosis of tension-type headache depends on the diagnostic criteria and method. As such, the actual prevalence of patients with headache may be much higher than believed.

2. Basic concept of traditional Oriental medicine

Traditional Oriental medicine is based on "Yin" and "Yang" and the "Five Elements Theory" [4, 5]. "Yin" and "Yang" are mutually opposed, representing related aspects of objects and ideas, such as male and female, right and left, and morning and evening. The Five Elements Theory describes five elements: wood, fire, earth, metal, and water, with everything in the world belonging to one of these five elements. For example, the liver, heart, spleen, lungs, and kidneys fall under the elements of wood, fire, earth, metal, and water, respectively. Of note, the liver and heart in Oriental medicine are not the same as the liver and heart as understood in Western medicine; the liver controls the systemic blood flow and Qi. Qi is a transmutable energy in traditional Chinese medicine that is presumed to flow through 12 meridians in the body [6]. Functional damage to the liver subsequently induces headache and vertigo. The heart controls mental activity, such as memory and intelligence, as well as the tongue; therefore, heart dysfunction can cause taste and language dysfunction. The spleen controls the digestion and absorption of food from the stomach, so spleen dysfunction induces stomachache and diarrhea. The lungs control breathing, and the skin is a barrier against external chemicals and infection. Therefore, lung dysfunction results in catching a cold and respiratory dysfunction. The kidneys control vitality and are related to the ears, so kidney dysfunction can cause a number of diseases, chills, and hearing loss.

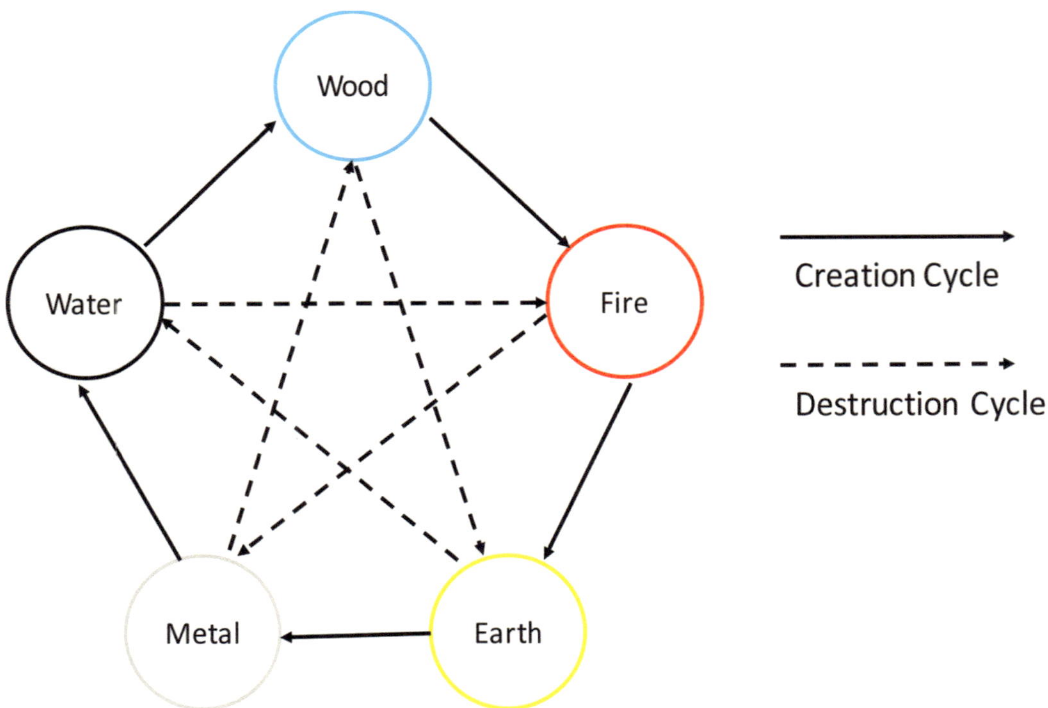

Figure 1. "Creation cycle" and "destruction cycle" (this figure is originally created by authors).

Additionally, the Five Elements Theory includes two relationships: the "creation cycle" and "destruction cycle" (**Figure 1**). The creation cycle is the "mother–child relationship," which repeats in circulation, and the destruction cycle occurs when one of the five elements wins against or limits another element [4]. Oriental medicine applies this theory for medical treatment and diagnosis. By maintaining balanced creation and destruction cycles, we can maintain good health. If those relationships become unbalanced, acupuncture and Chinese medicine are used to restore the balance.

3. The use of acupoints as a therapy for headache

Acupuncture has been used to treat various diseases, and there are many reports, from various countries around the world, on the use of acupuncture as a therapy for headaches. Acupuncture has been used to relieve tension-type headaches and prevent migraine attacks.

Finger cun (F-cun)	
1 F-cun	Thumb measurement: The width of the interphalangeal joint of the thumb is taken as 1 F-cun
	The distance between the ends of the two radial creases of the interphalangeal joints of the middle finger is taken as 1 F-cun when the thumb and the middle finger are flexed to form a circle
3 F-cun	Finger width measurement: when the index, middle, ring, and little fingers of the subject are extended and closed together, the width of the four fingers on the dorsal crease of the proximal interphalangeal joint of the middle finger is taken as 3 F-cun

Table 1. The finger-cun measurement methods (this table is originally created by authors based on Ref. [7]).

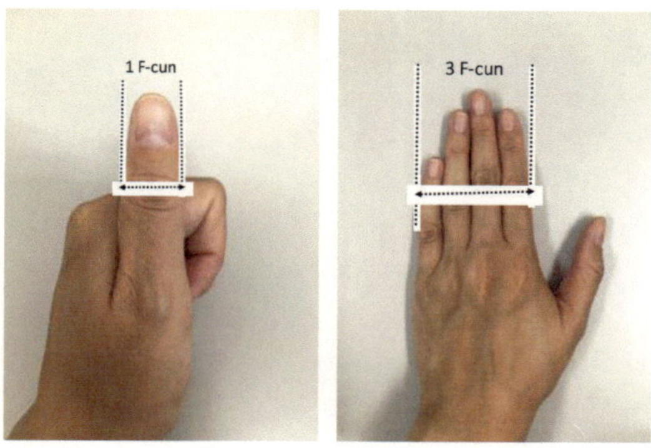

Figure 2. F-cun (this figure is originally created by authors).

Acupoints are determined using one of three typical methods [7]. The first is proportional bone (skeletal) cun (B-cun); this method divides the height of the human body into 75 equal units. Using joints on the surface of the body as the primary landmarks, the length and width of every body part are measured by such proportions [7]. Specifically, we divide the height of the human body into 75 equal units and then estimate the length and width of certain parts of the body based on such units. One unit is equal to 1 cun. B-cun is the most accurate method, as it measures each person's physical length, but it is complex. As such, other measurements are often used for convenience [7, 8] (**Table 1**). The second method is finger cun (F-cun), which uses a person's finger width to determine the acupuncture points (**Figure 2**). One B-cun and 1 F-cun are almost the same length. F-cun is determined using two methods. The first is thumb measurement using the width of the interphalangeal joints. Another is middle-finger cun (**Figure 3**). Middle-finger cun is the distance between the ends of the two radial creases of the interphalangeal joints of the middle finger is taken as 1 F-cun when the thumb and the middle finger are flexed to form a circle [7]. The last method is finger breadth, which uses the width of the distal phalanx of the middle finger to determine the acupuncture points (**Figure 4**). This method should not be confused with the middle finger cun. This method is rarely used. Given that all of these methods result in some degree of variation in acupuncture point determination.

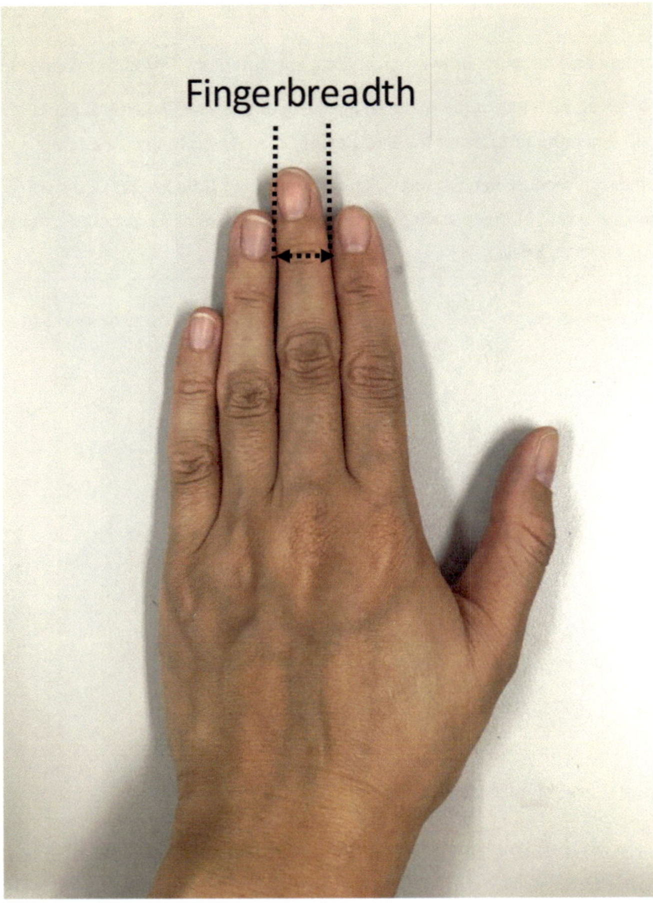

Figure 3. Middle-finger cun (this figure is originally created by authors).

10]).

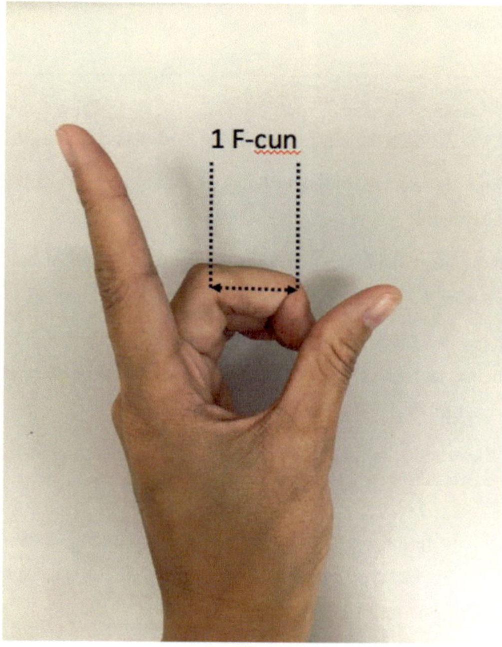

Figure 4. Finger breadth (this figure is originally created by authors).

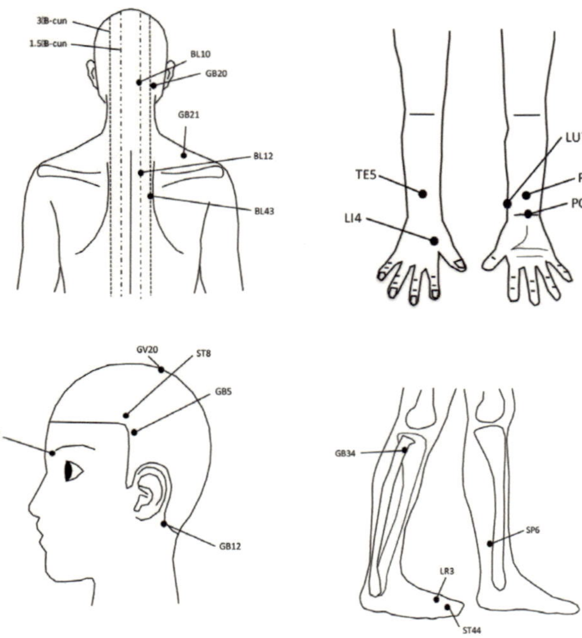

Figure 5. The acupoints used for the treatment of headache (this figure is originally created by authors based on Ref [9, 10]).

English name	Chinese name	Locations
Head region		
BL2	Cuanzhu	On the head, in the depression at the medial end of the eyebrow
GV20	Baihui	When the ears are folded, GV20 is located at the midpoint of the connecting line between the auricular apices
ST8	Touwei	On the head, 0.5 B-cun directly superior to the anterior hairline at the corner of the forehead, 4.5 B-cun lateral to the anterior median line
GB5	Xuanlu	On the head, at the midpoint of the curved line from ST8 to GB7 (on the head, at the junction of the vertical line of the posterior border of the temple hairline and the horizontal line of the apex of auricle)
GB12	Wangu	In the anterior region of the neck, in the depression posteroinferior to the mastoid process
Neck and back regions		
BL10	Tianzhu	In the posterior region of the neck, at the same level as the superior border of the spinous process of the second cervical vertebra (C2), in the depression lateral to the trapezius muscle
GB20	Fengchi	In the anterior region of the neck, inferior to the occipital bone, in the depression between the origins of sternocleidomastoid and the trapezius muscles
BL43	Gaohuang	In the upper back region, at the same level as the inferior border of the spinous process of the fourth vertebra (T4), 3 B-cun lateral to the posterior median line
GB21	Jianjing	In the posterior region of the neck, at the midpoint of the line connecting the spinous process of the seventh cervical vertebra (C7) with the lateral end of the acromion
BL12	Fengmen	In the upper back region, at the same level as the inferior border of the spinous process of the second thoracic vertebra (T2), 1.5 B-cun lateral to the posterior median line
Upper limbs		
LI4	Hegu	On the dorsum of the hand, radial to the midpoint of the second metacarpal bone
PC6	Neiguan	On the anterior aspect of the forearm, between the tendons of the Palmaris, longus and the flexor carpi radialis, 2 B-cun proximal to the wrist crease
TE5	Waiguan	On the posterior aspect of the forearm, midpoint of the interosseous space between the radius and the ulna, 2 B-cun proximal to the dorsal wrist crease
PC7	Daling	On the anterior aspect of the wrist, between the tendons of Palmaris longus and the flexor carpi radialis, on the palmar wrist crease
LU7	Lieque	On the radial aspect of the forearm, between the tendons of the abductor pollicis longus and the extensor pollicis brevis muscles, in the groove for the abductor pollicis longus tendon, 1.5 B-cun superior to the palmar wrist
Lower limbs		
SP6	Sanyinjiao	On the tibial aspect of the leg, posterior to the medial border of the tibia, 3 B-cun superior to the prominence of the medial malleulus

English name	Chinese name	Locations
LR3	Taichong	On the dorsum of the foot, between the first and second metatarsal bones, in the depression distal to the junction of the bases of the two bones, over the distals pedis artery
ST44	Neiting	On the dorsum of the foot, between the second and third toes, posterior to the web margin, at the border between the red and white flesh
GB34	Yanglingquan	On the fibular aspect of the leg, in the depression anterior and distal to the head of the fibula

Table 2. Acupuncture point locations (this table is originally created by authors based on Ref. [7]).

The acupoints used for the treatment of headaches are located on the upper trapezius muscle, the splenius muscle, the semispinal muscle, the levator scapulae muscle, and the rhomboids muscle. These include the bladder meridian, BL10; the gallbladder meridian, GB20, GB12, GB21, and BL43 and acupoints in the trigeminal regions, GB4, GB5, and GB6; the stomach meridian, ST8, ST6, and ST and the peripheral limbs; the large intestine meridian, LI4; the liver meridian, LR3; and the triple energizer meridian, TE5, GB34, and others (**Figure 5**, **Table 2**) [7, 9, 10]. The acupoints in the neck and back regions are suitable for electro-acupuncture (EA).

4. Reports of acupuncture as a therapy for headaches

In patients with migraine without aura, the number of headache attacks and analgesic use among patients who received acupuncture were significantly decreased in comparison with those who were treated with flunarizine [11].

Kikuchi et al. reported the effects of acupuncture on headache. They examined the numbers of medication days and headache days using a headache diary and found that the number of days in patients who experienced migraines, chronic tension-type headache, medication overuse headache, and chronic migraines decreased by 75, 50, 30, and 20%, respectively [12].

Thus, the effects of acupuncture differed according to the diagnosis. Yamaguchi et al. evaluated the effects of acupuncture in patients with tension-type headache using plethysmography, electromyography, and thermography [13]. Acupuncture was found to be effective for treating headaches because it normalized the excess tension of the neck and upper shoulder muscles rather than the head muscles [13]. However, few articles have classified headaches in detail and examined the effectiveness of acupuncture. Thus, there is no clear evidence of the types of headache for which acupuncture is effective or whether acupuncture should be performed in the attack phase or intermittent phase. Acupuncture therapy is classified as a Grade B treatment in the Japanese clinical practice guideline for chronic headache, which was published by the Japanese Society of Neurology and Headache in 2013 [14].

A Cochrane review reported that there was no significant difference in the clinical effects of true acupuncture and sham acupuncture, but that the number of headache days was decreased by the intervention [15]. Acupuncture was reported to be more effective and to be associated with fewer side effects than preventive medications [9].

A large clinical study of acupuncture for headache was conducted in the European Union. The number of headache days at 3 months after acupuncture significantly decreased from 8.4 to 4.7 days in the acupuncture group, while it decreased from 8.1 to 7.5 days in controls. In the economic study, acupuncture improved the quality of life and was highly cost-effective [16]. The placebo effect of acupuncture, however, is reported to be nearly 40% [17]. The accurate effect should be verified by a double-blind controlled trial, but it is difficult to establish control groups in acupuncture studies.

Acupuncture studies are associated with another problem with regard to the reproducibility of the treatment. In most reports, acupuncture was performed by an experienced acupuncturist; however, many parts depend on the technique of operator.

The accurate effect should be verified by a double-blind controlled trial, but it is difficult to establish control groups in acupuncture studies. So, some studies have used objective assessments. Chassot et al. reported a crossover trial regarding the effect of electro-acupuncture (EA) on chronic tension-type headache, including an assessment using a biological sample [17]. The visual analog scale score decreased more than 50% following EA in nine patients, but it also decreased in the sham period for five patients. The serum brain-derived neurotrophic factor was inversely correlated with pain intensity and degree of depression.

Kinfe et al. recently reported that presurgical acupuncture predict the effect of surgical occipital nerve stimulation (ONS) [18]. Twelve patients with chronic refractory headache syndrome eligible for ONS were treated using EA (100 Hz, 30 min) before ONS. For EA, four needles were inserted subcutaneously at the level of C1, defined as 3 cm below the occipital protuberance, 1.5 cm bilateral from the midline (two needles), and 3.5 cm bilateral from the midline (two needles), to ensure that it reached the occipital afferent distribution area [18]. The results showed that surgically implanted ONS was effective in some patients who had previously been non-responsive to acupuncture. Acupuncture may be a useful new tool for presurgical assessment.

5. Imaging studies of acupuncture for the treatment of headaches

Some recent reports have assessed the objective effects as well as the subjective effects of acupuncture in the treatment of headaches. Quirico et al. reported that acupuncture altered the cerebral blood flow [19]. The mean cerebral blood flow was changed by the acupoints.

Functional MRI (fMRI) is a form of objective imaging study. Recently, a study was performed to investigate brain dysfunction in patients with migraine and chronic tension-type headache [20]. In the study of the pain-induced activation of fMRI, migraine patients demonstrated specific brain activation in the interictal period in comparison with controls. The regions that were activated included the temporal pole, the parahippocampal gyrus, anterior cingulate cortex, lentiform nuclei, fusiform gyrus, subthalamic nucleus, hippocampus, middle cingulate cortex, somatosensory cortex, and the dorsolateral prefrontal cortex. Decreased activation was observed at the secondary somatosensory cortex, precentral gyrus, superior temporal gyrus, and the brainstem. The findings differed in the interictal, ictal, and preictal phases. Many fMRI studies have suggested the imbalance of the facilitation and inhibition of the pain signal conduction effect hypersensitivity in migraine.

In Japan, Yamaguchi et al. reported a change in the cerebral blood flow in migraine patients before and after acupuncture using arterial spin-labeled MRI [21]. Before acupuncture, the cerebral blood flow in migraine patients was high in the occipital and right temporal lobes and low at the left temporal and parietal lobes in comparison with controls. After acupuncture, a specific increase was observed in the cerebral blood flow of the thalamus, hypothalamus, pars opercularis, and insula of migraine patients.

Li et al. treated patients with migraine without aura with standard acupuncture five times per week during a 4-week period and examined the pain score and resting-state fMRI [22]. Patients with migraine without aura were found to have decreased functional connectivity in the left precentral gyrus, postcentral gyrus, left supramarginal gyrus, and the lower left parietal lobe. Furthermore, they found that the decreases in these functions were improved by the acupuncture therapy.

We hypothesize that acupuncture affects not only peripheral circulation, but also central nervous function. However, few scientific studies have investigated the effects of acupuncture for headache by assessing cerebral function. In the future, an objective clinical study assessing the effect of acupuncture on headache should be conducted.

Author details

Sumire Chiku[1] and Yasushi Shibata[2*]

*Address all correspondence to: yshibata@md.tsukuba.ac.jp

1 Graduate School of Comprehensive Human Sciences, University of Tsukuba, Tsukuba, Ibaraki, Japan

2 Department of Neurosurgery, Mito Medical Center, Headache Clinic, Mito Kyodo General Hospital, University of Tsukuba, Tsukuba, Ibaraki, Japan

References

[1] Global Burden of Disease Study 2013 Collaborators. Global, regional, and national incidence, prevalence, and years lived with disability for 301 acute and chronic diseases and injuries in 188 countries, 1990–2013: a systematic analysis for the Global Burden of

Disease Study 2013. Lancet (London, England). 2015;386(9995):743–800. doi:10.1016/S0140-6736(15)60692-4

[2] Bebbington P. The World Health Report 2001. Social Psychiatry and Psychiatric Epidemiology. 2001;36(10):473–474. doi:10.1007/s001270170010

[3] Stovner LJ, Hagen K, Jensen R, Katsarava Z, Lipton R, Scher AI, Steiner TJ and Zwart J-A. The global burden of headache: a documentation of headache prevalence and disability worldwide. Cephalalgia. 2007;27(3):193–210. doi:10.1111/j.1468-2982.2007.01288.x

[4] Omura Y. Acupuncture Medicine. Tokyo: Japan Publications, Inc.; 1996.

[5] Kyokasho shippitsu shoiinkai, Japan College Association of Oriental Medicine (Eds.). Oriental Medicine Outline. Kanagawa, Japan: IDO NO NIPPON SHA; 2009 (in Japanese, author translation).

[6] Cady R, Farmer K. Acupuncture in the treatment of headache: a traditional explanation of an ancient art. Headache. 2015;55(3):457–464. doi:10.1111/head.12523

[7] WHO Regional Office for the Western Pacific (Eds.). WHO Standard Acupuncture Point Locations in the Western Pacific Region. Geneva, Switzerland: World Health Organization; 2013.

[8] Japan Association of Massage and Acupuncture Teachers (Eds.). New Edition Meridian-Acupuncture Point Outline. Kanagawa, Japan: IDO NO NIPPON SHA; 2013 (in Japanese, author translation).

[9] Linde K, Allais G, Brinkhaus B, Manheimer E, Vickers A, White A. Acupuncture for migraine prophylaxis. Cochrane Database of Systemetic Reviews. 2011;21(1):1–87. doi:10.1002/14651858.CD001218.pub2.Acupuncture

[10] Linde K, Allais G, Brinkhaus B, Manheimer E, Vickers A, White A. Acupuncture for tension-type headache. The Cochrane Database of Systematic Reviews. 1996;(1):1–44. doi:10.1002/14651858.CD007587

[11] Allais G, De Lorenzo C, Quirico P, Airola G, Tolardo G, Mana O, Benedetto C. Acupuncture in the prophylactic treatment of migraine without aura: a comparison with flunarizine. Headache. 2002;42(9):855–861. doi:10.1046/j.1526-4610.2002.02203.x

[12] Kikuchi T, Yamaguchi S. Effect of acupuncture for migraine and tension-type headache to request to specialists. Gendai Shinkyu-Gaku. 2014;14:111–118 (in Japanese, author translation).

[13] Yamaguchi S. Analgesic effects of oriental medicine (acupuncture and moxibustion) on headache (II). The Journal of The Japanese Society of Balneology, Climatology and Physical Medicine 1987;50(4):220–231.

[14] Japanese Society of Neurology and Headache. Clinical Practice Guideline for Chronic Headache. Tokyo, Japan: Igakushoin; 2013 (in Japanese).

[15] Da Silva A. Acupuncture for migraine prevention. Headache: The Journal of Head and Face Pain. 2015;55:470–473. doi:10.1111/head.12525

[16] Witt C, Reinhold T, Jena S, Brinkhaus B, Willich S.N. Cost-effectiveness of acupuncture treatment in patients with headache. Cephalalgia. 2008;28(4):334–345. doi:10.1111/j.1468-2982.2007.01504.x

[17] Chassot M, Dussan-Sarria J, Sehn F, Deitos A, de Souza A, Vercelino R, Torres I, Fregni F, Caumo W. Electroacupuncture analgesia is associated with increased serum brain-derived neurotrophic factor in chronic tension-type headache: a randomized, sham controlled, crossover trial. BMC Complementary and Alternative Medicine. 2015; 15:144–154. doi:10.1186/s12906-015-0664-x

[18] Kinfe T, Pintea B, Roeske S, Guresir A, Guresir E, Vatter H. Percutaneous nerve field stimulation (PENS) of the occipital region as a possible predictor for occipital nerve stimulation (ONS) responsiveness in refractory headache disorders? A feasibility study. Cephalalgia: An International Journal of Headache. 2016;36(8):779–789. doi: 10.1177/0333102415613765

[19] Quirico P, Allais G, Ferrando M, De Lorenzo C, Burzio C, Bergandi F, Rolando S, Schiapparelli P, Benedetto C. Effects of the acupoints PC 6 Neiguan and LR 3 Taichong on cerebral blood flow in normal subjects and in migraine patients. Neurological Sciences: Official Journal of the Italian Neurological Society and of the Italian Society of Clinical Neurophysiology. 2014;35(Suppl 1):129–133. doi:10.1007/s10072-014-1754-0

[20] Schwedt T, Chiang C, Chong C, Dodick D. Functional MRI of migraine. The Lancet Neurology. 2015;14(1):81–91. doi:10.1016/S1474-4422(14)70193-0

[21] Yamaguchi S, Araki N, Matsuda H. Cerebral blood flow assessment before and after acupuncture using arterial spin labeled MRI. Journal of Saitama Medical School. 2012;39(1):39–40 (in Japanese, author translation).

[22] Li K, Zhang Y, Ning Y, Zhang H, Liu H, Fu C, Ren Y, Zou Y. The effects of acupuncture treatment on the right frontoparietal network in migraine without aura patients. The Journal of Headache and Pain. 2015;16(33):1–10. doi:10.1186/s10194-015-0518-4